Pharmacy Preregistration Handbook

Pharmacy Preregistration Handbook

A survival guide

Second edition

Lindsay Taylor

BSc(Pharm), MA, MRPharmS

Clinical Governance and NHS Information Manager
Lloyds Pharmacy
Coventry, UK

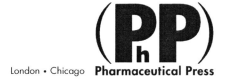

London • Chicago **Pharmaceutical Press**

An imprint of RPS Publishing

1 Lambeth High Street, London SE1 7JN, UK
100 South Atkinson Road, Suite 206, Grayslake, Il 60030-7820, USA

© Pharmaceutical Press 2002

RPS Publishing is the wholly-owned publishing organisation of the
Royal Pharmaceutical Society of Great Britain

First edition 2000
Second edition 2002
Reprinted 2006

Text design by Barker/Hilsdon, Lyme Regis, Dorset
Typeset by Type Study, Scarborough, North Yorkshire
Printed in Great Britain by CPI Antony Rowe, Eastbourne

ISBN-10 0 85369 513 X
ISBN-13 978 0 85369 513 4

A catalogue record for this book is available from the British Library

Contents

Preface

As a preregistration trainee you will have received a daunting amount of printed information detailing what you are expected to be able to do by the end of the year. A large plastic wallet from the Royal Pharmaceutical Society of Great Britain containing two looseleaf folders will probably have been supplemented by even more material from your employer. Tutors (and trainees) will also be aware of other resources – such as textbooks and distance learning packages – that need to be utilised in order to fulfil all the requirements for registration.

Inevitably, there are many questions from those undertaking the programme – regarding the structure of the year, the syllabus, the performance standards and most especially the exam – just to mention a few. It is not difficult to envisage situations that could develop into major problems if satisfactory solutions are not found quickly.

Tutors (especially anyone taking on the onerous responsibility for the first time) may also feel overwhelmed by the sheer volume of paper that they are expected to read, assimilate and act upon – all in the course of a busy working day. Many of those involved know that the answers to most of the commonly asked questions are to be found in the resources mentioned – somewhere. However, for every preregistration trainee and/or tutor to research each query individually takes a great deal of time and effort; for some the task is overwhelming. Those who lack the requisite ability to organise themselves are often the students who relied on the university system and friends for survival, and are possibly now working in a situation where they are isolated from other trainees. The preregistration year may be spent finding the answers to problems generated by a lack of appropriate organisational skills, instead of concentrating on acquiring knowledge of, and developing competence in, the skills vital for practice as a pharmacist. For many who are in such a position, the consequence is not being able to meet the exacting criteria for registration – including of course reaching the required standard in the exam.

The *Pharmacy Preregistration Handbook: A survival guide* 2nd edition is intended to enable everyone involved in the preregistration training programme to concentrate on maximising opportunities to create – and benefit from – a wide variety of appropriate learning activities. The first chapter deals with minor and major issues that may hinder the process; common problems, including those associated with the workplace-based training programme, are discussed in some detail. However, the *survival guide* does not – and indeed cannot – provide the answer to every query; instead, it is designed to help trainees, and their tutors, find the solution for themselves by accessing the appropriate primary reference source effectively and efficiently.

The nature of the registration examination is a cause of great concern to trainees and their tutors, who agree that many problems are generated by its unique demands. Even graduates who have been successful in previous examinations are quite naturally very concerned at their ability to overcome the final hurdle before their hard work can be put into (pharmacy) practice. In many cases, the fears are due to perceptions of the exam being different from the others that they have taken – which, of course, is correct; it is intended to assess the application of knowledge and cognitive skills necessary for practice as a pharmacist, not those of a science graduate. The need to perform calculations accurately without a calculator under examination conditions, and the demands of problem-solving, practice-based questions are the most common sources of anxiety. Chapters 2, 3 and 4 are therefore devoted to learning activities, including some suggested by successful candidates, which will enable others to prepare and revise appropriately. In Chapter 5 new questions, together with suggested answers and explanations, allow preregistration trainees to practise what they have learnt.

It is important to add, before too many tutors and trainees quite rightly hasten to point it out, that the registration exam is the culmination of a year of intensive training in the practice of the profession of pharmacy. The student who has worked diligently throughout the year should have no qualms about their ability to meet the challenges of the examination and of registration. Chapter 6 allows preregistration trainees to reflect very briefly on what they have accomplished during the year, and to begin to plan their further development as a practising pharmacist.

This last paragraph is addressed specifically to preregistration trainees: as graduates, you are undoubtedly only too aware that the onus and responsibility for your learning experience is now firmly on you. The fundamental goal of the book is therefore to help you access and understand the multitude of information with which you are presented in order to help everyone involved in the training process achieve the registration of a competent trainee. May you soon be pharmacists.

Lindsay Taylor
October 2001

Acknowledgements

I would like to thank the many preregistration trainees, tutors and colleagues at Lloydspharmacy with whom I have worked for their invaluable ideas and contributions. I very much hope the readers of the *survival guide* will learn from their experiences, and that the profession of pharmacy will benefit as a result.

Thanks are also due to my long-suffering husband, Gerald (Prince), for his constructive advice, and for his continued devotion to the sports channels whilst I was otherwise occupied.

About the author

Lindsay Taylor studied pharmacy at City of Leicester Polytechnic (now De Montfort University), after several years working as a dispensing assistant and laboratory technician.

Her extensive experience of community pharmacy practice, and eight years teaching science in a secondary school, led to her appointment as one of the first community-based Boots' teacher-practitioners at De Montfort University, Leicester in 1990. The post involved teaching pharmacy law, ethics, dispensing, and many other aspects of pharmacy practice. She was also a module leader, a member of the team responsible for implementing the Post Graduate Diploma in Community Clinical Pharmacy, and the chair of the staff-student consultative committee. In addition to teaching, she acted as a supervisor to many undergraduates undertaking research projects, several of which have been presented at British Pharmaceutical Conferences. In 1997 she gained a Master of Arts in Learning and Teaching for research that involved measuring the quality of pharmacy practice.

At Boots she was responsible for the organisation and delivery of many aspects of the company preregistration programme, including working with individual students and those who failed the registration exam.

In 1997 she co-authored (with Gordon E Appelbe and Joy Wingfield) *Practical Exercises in Pharmacy Law and Ethics* which presents teaching exercises that enable undergraduates and pre-registration trainees to develop a problem-solving approach to the understanding of pharmacy law and ethics. That book has also been updated recently.

Lindsay became NHS Information and Services Manager at the Head Office of Lloydspharmacy in 1999, where she is involved in researching and evaluating many aspects of NHS policy. In January 2002 her role expanded to include responsibility for clinical governance throughout the Company.

Notes on the text

The following phrases, shortened terms and icons have been used throughout the *Handbook*. You may find it useful to familiarise yourself with the adopted terminology before reading the chapters.

Byelaws	RPSGB Byelaws on Preregistration Training: Section XX of the manual
CBTP	Competence-based training programme
Exam Regulations	Regulations for the Royal Pharmaceutical Society's Registration Examination
Journal	*The Pharmaceutical Journal*
manual	RPSGB Preregistration Training Manual
Medicines, Ethics and Practice guide (MEP)	*Medicines, Ethics and Practice: A guide for pharmacists*
Society	The Royal Pharmaceutical Society of Great Britain
	Indicates the question is from a closed-book paper (Paper 1)
	Indicates the question is from an open-book paper (Paper 2)

Abbreviations

BNF	*British National Formulary*
CBTP	competence-based training programme
CD	Controlled Drug
CPPE	Centre for Postgraduate Pharmacy Education
FAQ	frequently asked question
GP	general practitioner
GSL	general sale list
IMS	industrial methylated spirits
MEP	*Medicines, Ethics and Practice: A guide for pharmacists*
NPA	National Pharmaceutical Association
NSAID	non-steroidal anti-inflammatory drug
OTC	over the counter (medicines)
P	pharmacy-only (medicine)
POM	prescription-only medicine
RPSGB	Royal Pharmaceutical Society of Great Britain
TPAP	Training Performance Assessment Programme

1

The 'problem pages'

1.1 Introduction

Preregistration trainees are sent a great deal of written information by the Royal Pharmaceutical Society of Great Britain (RPSGB); it is probable that your employer has also added to the pile of papers stacked in a corner of your bedroom. Somewhere you will undoubtedly have the answer to most of the commonly asked questions concerning the administrative details of the preregistration year. It is also possible that you have had the benefit of courses designed to develop the interpersonal skills necessary to equip you with the means to handle the practical issues that arise when dealing with the public. Why, then, is there a complete chapter on problems? Doesn't it just repeat the same material? The answer to that question, and the justification for the chapter, lies in the following paragraphs.

If you read ahead, you will find that the answers to questions are not repeated; instead, you are usually referred to the entry in your official RPSGB Preregistration Training material. For the preregistration trainees following the new performance assessment programme, this now consists of looseleaf plastic folders containing the sheets that make up your Workbook and Portfolio. However, for at least the next two or three years it will not be possible for everyone to follow every aspect of the new programme, due to difficulties arranging sufficient cross-sector training placements, which are a significant feature of the new performance assessment. A number of trainees will therefore still be using a 'manual' as the source of their training and reference material. However, it, too, has been radically changed and contains the great majority of the resources sent to those following the new programme, since it was felt that preregistration trainees would be disadvantaged if they could not access the same updated and

improved material. The basic differences between the two programmes (and hence the contents of the folder and the manual) are
in the layout and presentation of the two resources, and in the standards by which the workplace-based competence of the trainee is
assessed by their tutor. The new Training Performance Assessment
Programme (TPAP) contains Performance Standards which can
only be met by undertaking appropriate practice-based activities in
both community and hospital pharmacy. The sector-specific Competence Based Training Programme (CBTP) uses performance or
behavioural indicators to describe competence; the details of each
are in the tutees Workbook or the manual respectively. In order not
to confuse everyone too much by covering details of both alterna-
tives in one sentence, the 'Pharmacy Preregistration Handbook
2nd edition' will refer to the requirements of the new TPAP[1] programme. The number written in superscript refers to the summary
in Section 1.9.2 which draws together all the alternative references
to be used for those following the CBTP; refer to the number given
for the one that is appropriate to your placement. In the first year
of the new programme many trainees were confused as to which
scheme they were following and consequently received the wrong
material – check with your tutor.

The details of all aspects of the programme are contained in
the workbook[2], which has lots of information and activities; the
portfolio[2] has the vital forms and various other templates but is
otherwise empty, as it will also be used to store the 'evidence' that
you collect. Both folders are vital to the TPAP[1] and will be referred
to frequently.

However, having explained some of the complications associated with the changes, to return to the original question – why
bother making hard-pressed trainees go back to their folders[2] –
why not just respond to the question directly? After all, most
people find it easier to ask someone rather than find out for themselves, so why make life even harder? For a variety of important
reasons – the main one being that the original answer is correct;
repetition may omit a vital detail – and then who will be at fault?
As with all evidence, it is best to go to the primary source.

Further justification for the approach lies with a fundamental concept of teaching and learning – that active participation (where an individual invests time and effort) has a much better chance of being understood and acted upon. In other words, the intention is to help you to help yourself, and to provide assistance in the somewhat daunting process of finding the answer. In the pages that follow, you are therefore referred to the appropriate section in your workbook (or manual), which contains the RPSGB Byelaws on Preregistration Training (*Byelaws*) and the Regulations for the Royal Pharmaceutical Society's Registration Examination (*Exam Regulations*), instead of someone else's interpretation of a complicated situation.

Perhaps it is also a good time to clarify one or two points for the many dedicated pharmacists who have acted as tutors before, and haven't yet had time to get to grips with some of the issues raised in connection with the revised programme and why they were thought to be necessary. Table 1.1, which summarises many of the general differences, is presented on p. 4. It is not intended to be a comprehensive evaluation of the changes and the reasons for them, but to provide an overview of the most important features, especially necessary as many trainees will still be following the CBTP.

The rest of the chapter deals with the many problems with which everyone who is involved with preregistration trainees is familiar. The questions concerning administrative procedures that are asked – in spite of the information being readily available – are answered in Section 1.2 below. In order to ascertain the full range of problems that arise, the Education Division at the RPSGB, other organisations and individuals responsible for training were asked to contribute their 'Frequently Asked Questions' (FAQs). The twice-yearly bulletins sent to trainees and the Workbook both contain the official answers to many FAQs; this guide addresses some of the same issues – and a few new ones – in a little more detail. The collection of 'evidence' poses many problems for preregistration trainees and their tutors, so it is considered in Section 1.3. The many questions concerned with the exact details of entering for the examination, and its organisation, are considered in Section 1.4, and the procedure for registration in Section 1.5.

Table 1.1 To compare aspects of the old and revised preregistration programmes

(a) General points

	Previous programme and material	Revised programme and material	Comments regarding reasons etc.
1 Aim of programme (the term programme is used to indicate both the exam and the learning that takes place in the workplace, which is assessed separately)	To take the newly-graduated (or sandwich course student/overseas pharmacist) through a process of development to a point at which s/he is able to function as an independent professional practitioner	To make the transition from student to an effective member of pharmacy profession	Changes in response to meet the demands of the 'new NHS' – ■ More patient-focused ■ Removes barriers between sectors ■ More emphasis on professional behaviour and the interpersonal skills necessary for practice
2 Definition and details of 'competence' (the term used to demonstrate that the graduate meets the workplace-based assessment criteria)	The ability to perform consistently at the required standard Outcome not process important Performance to date must indicate consistency Not graded; either reaches the required standard or it doesn't – yet	Having the necessary skills, knowledge and attitudes to undertake the role of the pharmacist properly and consistently	'Competence', 'competencies' and other terminology such as behavioural indicators a nightmare for those unfamiliar with such concepts
3 Measurement of competence (to work towards 'proving' by providing evidence)	Professional and practical units that contain several elements, each containing detailed Performance Criteria – which may be further clarified by definitions – that formed the basis of the 13, 26 and 39-week appraisals	Performance standards and detailed indicators describe what the preregistration trainee is expected to be able to do; three-monthly assessments are supplemented by cumulative summaries	As it has proven difficult to arrange sufficient cross – sectorial placements to allow all the 2001 trainees to undertake the new programme, both measurement systems will be in operation. It is hoped that the situation will have been resolved by 2003
4 Exam pass criteria	70% overall	70% overall, including the calculations section	Applies to all preregistration trainees, regardless of programme followed

continued overleaf

	Previous programme and material	Revised programme and material	Comments regarding reasons etc.
5 A personal overall impression of trainees' training material	One huge folder (the manual) with masses of forms and important information that was difficult to carry about and access. Many students relied on further material from employers and tutors' explanations to know where to start	Much improved presentation, which should ensure that trainees have a clearer vision of the overall programme and what is expected of them – supported by the learning contract. The various activities provide a clear framework of support	Looseleaf format of Workbook and Portfolio[2] (for students) and workbook and information file[2] for tutors will mean that updates can be inserted in the appropriate place as they are received. The framework of essential activities for both should ensure that every graduate has the same opportunities, whichever programme they are following
6 A personal overall impression of tutors' material	Access to some parts of programme relied on compulsory attendance at RPSGB seminar. Undertaking initial tasks – such as assessing learning styles – was difficult to arrange for all new tutors, especially if they took over during the year	Clear indication of expectations regarding tutors' input from CPD/self assessment and agreement to tutor document. Contains all the material needed in the two tutors' folders – the Information file and Workbook[2]	

(b) Points regarding the changes to the tutor's role

	Previous programme and material	Revised programme and material	Comments regarding reasons etc.
1 Role, responsibilities, and desirable attributes of tutor (not comprehensive)	■ Acting as a willing, positive, role model, coach, mentor, learning resource, communicating with others involved in the programme to ensure sufficient skills and knowledge of programme etc. ■ Adhering to RPSGB standards for preregistration training, liaison and communication with RPSGB and others, evaluating implementation and effectiveness of programme, deciding on tutees' competence and suitability for registration	The new programme provides a very clear framework to ensure that the tutor understands exactly how and when to undertake the activities necessary to develop the appropriate personal skills to meet the development needs of every tutee (Many tutors will of course have had experience, both as part of their involvement as a tutor and as a normal part of their work in coaching and mentoring, for example. The assessment of developmental needs allows for	Although the role, responsibilities and desirable attributes are clearly stated in the original programme, and have not changed in the new one, experience has shown that there have been occasions (often beyond their control) where tutors have fallen short of the ideal, which has had adverse effects for the trainee. The formal agreement to tutor document and learning contract provide an evidence base to refer to in the event of any problems It's important to keep copies; hopefully, if

continued overleaf

Table 1.1 (continued)

	Previous programme and material	Revised programme and material	Comments regarding reasons etc.
	■ Having sufficient availability, accessibility, experience and personal and professional commitment to ensure the success of the programme and the trainee	different levels of experience and individual CPD needs)	the tutor and tutee have read and act upon all the advice and new frameworks in place, there will be no need to refer to them again
2 Role of other pharmacists/trainers in the programme	A bit muddled – it was accepted that it was not always the tutor who had day-to-day supervision, especially in large hospital pharmacies, but how much other 'trainers' could do wasn't clear	Very clear overview regarding the different roles of tutor, Mentor, Managers is presented in the Tutor Information pack[2]	Possible changes to the byelaws are envisaged to encompass supervision of a number of tutees in a large establishment

(c) Points regarding the changes from the tutee's perspective

	Previous programme and material	Revised programme and material	Comments regarding reasons etc.
1 Role, responsibilities and desirable attributes of preregistration trainees – again not comprehensive, and, of course, to be developed throughout the year to meet performance standards/behavioural criteria	Less emphasis on recognising and developing their own preferred learning style; coaching consisted of steering the tutee	Responsibility firmly placed with tutee to ensure that they understand the key element of the programme is EXPERIENCE of all activities Basically a trainee who: ■ takes responsibility for their own learning and plans their own progress development and learning activities ■ prepares and organises themselves and their evidence prior to meetings ■ enthusiastically takes every opportunity to learn, and ■ applies their theoretical knowledge to practice, will endear themselves to all concerned in their development. ■ Using a variety of learning techniques, including a problem-solving approach, is especially appropriate to present and future practice, and is reflected in the type of questions set in the registration exam	Changes reflected in move from a syllabus for the programme which was divided into those skills needed in practice and different ones for exam; in the new one they are seen as inextricably linked. Focus on developing professional behaviour, self-management and patient focus in order to demonstrate behaviours in practice. Implicit within practical learning and tested by exam

Some of the more complex problems, which are often difficult for individual trainees to solve, have been addressed in Section 1.6. The topics have arisen as the result of anonymous questionnaires completed by a variety of preregistration trainees and their tutors. As it is impossible to provide definitive answers for every situation, the emphasis is on a general approach. For example, the questions do not cover the specific information applicable to 'sandwich' course students or to overseas pharmacists. Some additional activities are also included to provide preregistration trainees with initial ideas of how to tackle issues such as being sufficiently assertive to enable them to progress in their learning.

All the questions raised are presented in the format of a possible/actual problem and its suggested solution, and are organised into a chronological order as far as possible. Even if a particular difficulty has not been covered, the principles for seeking further help should enable you to have a better understanding of where suitable information can be found.

So, if your problem is organising yourself, losing bits of paper, relying on others too much, and/or a lack of confidence, don't worry – advice is at hand! Read on for lots of 'self-help' ideas on a wide variety of topics. Alternatively, if you know only too well what you want to do, but are having difficulty persuading others to contribute, there are some ideas for that situation too.

1.2 General administrative problems

I'm sure I should have done something more than agree on a starting date with my tutor – what?

Quite a lot actually! A question such as this one serves to illustrate several points:

- You are quite correct in thinking that the onus for your progress is on you – well done for getting that far. Now go back to the information pack that you were sent by the RPSGB during your final year at university. In previous years, a speaker visited all final year undergraduates, but in 1998–99 the procedure changed and a substantial pack of information is now distributed to all students. (NB the procedure for students taking a sandwich course is different, and will be dealt with by the university.) The pack includes a vital piece of paper known as 'the notification form for preregistration training'. If you don't have a form, contact the Education Division at the RPSGB (the Society) as soon as possible. Your training period will not be recognised by the Society until they have received this completed form from you. Send it back at least eight weeks before you intend to start work. Another point to remember is the limitation imposed on the dates when you can begin your training, which is to ensure that you have completed the statutory number of weeks (45) before taking the registration examination. See *Byelaw 26* for details.

- In addition to the completion of all forms on time, it is also vital that the accompanying fees are sent, or you will not receive your folders[2] of training material from the Society. As they contain all the necessary forms and information, you will be at a serious disadvantage if you have to start work without them.
- Perhaps this is also a suitable time to ensure that other procedures that need to take place prior to the preregistration year have been complied with. Briefly, the premises need to have been approved for preregistration training, and your tutor has to fulfil the requirements of the Society for preregistration training (*Byelaws 6–12*). There is also the 'agreement to tutor' document which is his/her part of the learning agreement between you, and the 'learning contract' to be filled in by both of you.
- In addition to getting a starting date and sorting out all the associated administration, it would also be in order to enquire about your contract of employment and working conditions. That means things like how many hours per week you will

work, and when your day off will be. You should be given a formal contract; if not, try to get everything in writing.

I'm not very good at organising bits of paper, but I know they're important this year. Which are essential – and what do I have to do with them?

Many students (and others) depend on their better-organised colleagues/parents/partners to get them to exams and other important life events on time and with the correct equipment. It is a habit that starts in early childhood, and if parents weren't so 'helpful', it could be abolished before going to university, to the benefit of all concerned. Others seem to be disorganised but just manage to elude punishment and the awful recriminations that follow when a vital deadline is missed. The more responsible souls will have learnt from past experiences, and will have bought themselves a *Filofax*, a diary or at least a notebook – and use it! It is unlikely that anyone in this category will need the following advice, which is for hopeless cases – those who, in spite of cumulative efforts by everyone involved, cannot conform to the rigid structure that has to be imposed for the complex system to work. So, if you are one of those who has finally realised that life is getting serious, and that you really need to get organised – read on. A major step has already been taken – you have read this section! What follows is not revolutionary – it's all in the workbook[2] – but just takes some finding. Start your planning now, before it's too late!

Some suggestions to help include:

○   Get a notebook/diary/*Dictaphone* that fits in your pocket and can be used as a day-to-day reminder about drugs to look up, tasks to complete, evidence to log, plans for the next appraisal etc.

○   Another useful tool would be a tray or drawer in an easily accessible place in the dispensary so that all the papers and journals that are sent to you can be put there for safekeeping before filing in your portfolio etc. Then, when you are searching for a vital form or piece of paper, there is at least a starting point at which to aim.

○ To help you in the future, every time you find some potentially useful information in your folders, index it with a *Post-it* note or even construct a proper, written index, so that you can find it again.

○ There is a useful summary of what happens to the various forms in the Portfolio[2]. The bulletins are also full of reminders about what is to be done – and when. Another useful resource is the checklist of expected mailings, customised for every type of trainee, to be found in the Workbook[2].

○ If you have a well organised friend, they may well agree to a system where they can help you with deadlines; no doubt they will have a weakness so you can repay the favour.

I really don't know whom I should ring first about my problem or where to find their number.

There may well be occasions when the only way to solve a problem is to phone someone – easy if you know the right person to contact and their number. However, if you don't, before worrying about whom to phone, think about who else a bit nearer home might be able – and willing – to help. The first person to approach, once you are sure that you cannot sort things out yourself, should be your tutor or someone else who works for the same organisation. In the new programme, it is quite possible that you will have other people with a specific role to play in your training. Their titles and responsibilities are described in the Workbook[2], together with examples of some other support mechanisms you may not have considered. However, not everyone is fortunate enough to have others able to help, or the problem may involve your tutor. The contact details for many of the sources of help are also listed in your workbook[2], although the recently introduced direct phone number to the preregistration training department (020 7572 2370) is not given. Don't forget to include your seven-digit number from the training record document sent to you in September if you do have to contact the Society. Another major change that has become obvious in the new programme is the use of email to contact the Society and the Internet to access a variety of resources. Although you may have had the appropriate facilities provided at university, that may not now be the case and is one more example of something you need to organise for yourself, or you will be disadvantaged.

I have always been healthy and am very rarely ill. Why do I have to go to the time and trouble – not to mention the possible cost – of obtaining a health declaration?

It is one of the prerequisites to registration that a health declaration is received with the examination entry. The medical examination must have taken place not more than 18 months before the anticipated date of registration. If the organisation for whom you are working does not organise a medical for you, then you will need to arrange to see either your general practitioner or another doctor registered in the UK to complete the health declaration form to be found in the Portfolio[2] – and they may charge a fee for doing so. There are many reasons why a potential pharmacist needs to prove that they are healthy. If you are going to be in sole charge of a pharmacy, you will be expected to be able to cope with the mental and physical demands that are engendered by the responsibility of the role. Another more pragmatic reason is the need to be able to resist the many germs that will be encountered as part of everyday life!

My tutor, with whom I've got on very well, is going on maternity leave. The new tutor is taking over next month. Do I have to contact the RPSGB?

Every year, there are a number of preregistration trainees who are affected to a greater or lesser extent by a change of tutor; the Society recognises the situation in *Byelaw 10*, which states that the establishment will still be registered for training for the rest of the year. However, as soon as you know about the change, you should complete the appropriate part of the 'Change of training details form' found in the Portfolio[2]. On the reverse side, the new tutor completes an undertaking (the 'Agreement to tutor' form) to the Society concerning their responsibilities, which should be followed up by a new learning contract, also to be found in the Portfolio[2], as soon as possible after they start. It will then be the new tutor's responsibility to assess their competence to meet the demands of acting as a tutor, and to plan their individual CPD accordingly. Before she goes, a wise step would be to check that your tutor has passed on as much information as possible about your progress so far, and that any assessments[3] already completed have been sent to the Society.

I have been ill and had to take two weeks off. Do I have to let the RPSGB know?

There are clear guidelines from the Society regarding absence through illness (*Byelaw 13*). You will need to contact the Education Division, who will inform the Registrar; any extension to your training will be at their discretion.

I can't find one of the essential texts that I must have – someone has thrown it away. Can I get a new one from the RPSGB?

The RPSGB cannot provide copies of any of the essential texts for the registration examination. The examination guidance notes and bulletin give a clear indication that it is the responsibility of potential candidates to identify and keep the relevant *British National Formulary* (BNF) and Drug Tariff when they are replaced. The Medicines, Ethics and Practice guide (MEP) is sent to all trainees with the *Pharmaceutical Journal* (the Journal). Details of the exact editions needed for the next examination are publicised in the Spring Bulletin prior to the next intake, so plenty of notice is given. Details are also given in the Workbook[2]. If you don't have the correct texts, and you answer a question wrongly, no credit can be given. Good bookshops either keep in stock, or can order, BNFs and MEPs at the retail price. Such an investment is probably worthwhile as soon as the edition becomes available, as you can then begin to practise using your customised copy in preparation for the exam.

Where do I get hold of CPPE packs – and which ones can I have?

The Centre for Postgraduate Pharmacy Education (CPPE) automatically sends to all preregistration trainees in England selected distance learning packages; for trainees in Wales and Scotland different arrangements apply. Details are given in the mailings list in the Workbook[2] and in the winter Bulletin.

Q *I'm a preregistration trainee working in an independent community pharmacy. My tutor recognises that it would be beneficial for me to meet and work with other trainees in my area. He has suggested that I organise a 'self-help' group, and that we choose our own agenda. Are there other similar groups, and if so, what suggestions might they make for making the best use of our time?*

A Assuming that the group is composed of other students in a similar position, the needs of the individuals concerned will dictate the agenda; there is certain to be at least one common topic, which would be a good starting point. Perhaps at the first meeting everyone could suggest three syllabus items that they would like to cover, with the premise that the most popular will be addressed first. Alternatively, if the group is mixed and has graduates from other areas of practice – for example, those at the local hospitals – there are many possibilities for the pooling of resources and expertise.

The difficulty most likely to arise is not what to study but how it can all be done. One possibility is for a small sub-group – say three trainees – to select a topic and research it, and then present their findings to the rest. It may be possible to use pharmaceutical companies to provide resources; the process of communication and persuasion would provide you with valuable evidence of several competencies! If you have been to local branch meetings with your tutor, it is probable that members may well have considerable expertise that they would be pleased to share with potential members of the profession – there's no harm in asking!

Other sessions could well be based on a particular clinical area – use the same order as in the BNF and practise finding doses, side-effects, interactions, etc. – or pooling information about resources that different members of the group have access to in their workplace. The main thing is to get together and use the time constructively, which probably means a bit of planning and preparation is called for – which could be another source of evidence.

Which reference books are supposed to be in the dispensary?

A list of essential and recommended reference sources is given in the examination syllabus; for each section, the text that is needed for the exam is supplemented by lots of other useful suggestions. Further relevant texts that become available during the year are listed in the bulletins.

How do I know which is the best book to use from those listed in the syllabus?

As a pharmacist one of the most vital skills you will need to demonstrate is the ability to know which resource to choose for each of the many queries encountered in the course of a working day. The ones that a pharmacist can be expected to know about range from the everyday – such as the BNF – to those which are used infrequently but of which they should be aware. In order to answer the original question, there is no substitute for learning by experience. Make sure you try to answer as many questions as possible without being told where to look for the necessary information. You should also get plenty of practice at using the three books needed for the 'open-book' part of the exam.

How do I know which book to buy to help me with a particular topic?

A further consideration, which is discussed in Chapter 3, is the need to have access to appropriate reference sources in order to prepare for the exam. As the needs of each student are very different, specific advice is inappropriate. A good idea would be to ask graduates from different schools of pharmacy, and to read the book reviews in the Journal.

What can I do to find the information I need faster?

The previous question referred to the need to use reference sources effectively – but efficiency is also important. You will not only be expected to use the most appropriate book, but also to find the information as quickly as possible – that is, efficiently. Try the 'turn to' test described below.

> Work with another preregistration trainee. The idea is for one to say 'turn to . . .,' and the other to find the necessary information quickly in one of the 'open-book' reference sources. Take turns – each person is bound to know about useful bits of information hidden away of which the other is not aware, and you will both gain practice in using the index quickly.

Some examples to get you started are:

- Turn to the section in the BNF that gives equivalent oral doses of the Controlled Drugs (CDs) morphine and diamorphine.
- Turn to the 'black list' in the *Drug Tariff.*
- Turn to the section in the MEP that summarises the CD regulations.

Someone told me the syllabus for the registration examination has changed quite a lot from last year. Why is this – was there anything wrong with the old one?

The exam syllabus is in your Workbook[2], and yes, you're quite right, it has changed – for some very good reasons which are outlined below. Incidentally, everyone will be taking the same registration exam, whichever performance assessment programme they follow.

The advent of the four-year degree has enabled a complete update of all aspects of undergraduate pharmacy courses to take place. The latest scientific advances and the sociological and ethical demands that are placed on all health professionals as a result must of course be reflected in any postgraduate courses such as the pre-registration programme. In addition, a vocational degree such as pharmacy will need to consider the demands of future employers such as the NHS as well as the current and future changes in professional practice.

The fundamental proposals for new ways of working encompassed in NHS policy are already being implemented by members of the profession, so it is vitally important that a training programme specifically designed to prepare you for practice as a pharmacist reflects those changes. Consequently, the exam syllabus and the other parts of the programme that prepares you to be a competent pharmacist have changed too. Many topics have been removed from the syllabus, and replaced by others that are more appropriate; one example is the theoretical aspects of sterilisation, which are covered in every undergraduate course. For anyone planning to work in the NHS, an understanding of the NHS concept of quality, clinical governance, is essential, and is given due prominence in the new syllabus. It will be very important to make sure you find out about such topics, which will probably not have been covered in sufficient detail - if at all - in undergraduate courses. You will find out more about how to interpret the exam syllabus and use the information it contains to your advantage in Chapter 5. You may be surprised to know that passing the exam and proving that you are competent are not the only conditions to be fulfilled before you are eligible to apply for registration as a pharmacist. An overview of all the requirements, including the necessity to follow one or other routes to competence, is presented in Fig. 1.1.

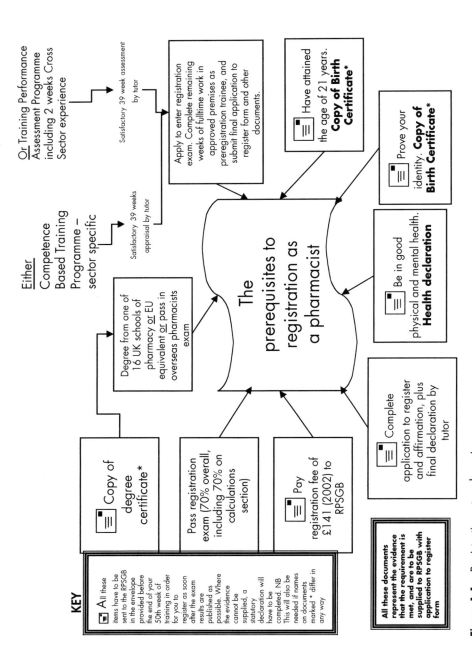

KEY

📄 All these items have to be sent to the RPSGB in the envelope provided before the the end of your 50th week of training in order for you to register as soon after the exam results are published as possible. Where the evidence cannot be supplied, a statutory declaration will have to be completed. NB This will also be needed if names on documents marked * differ in any way

Or Training Performance Assessment Programme including 2 weeks Cross Sector experience

Satisfactory 39 week assessment by tutor

Either Competence Based Training Programme – sector specific

Satisfactory 39 weeks appraisal by tutor

Apply to enter registration exam. Complete remaining weeks of fulltime work in approved premises as preregistration trainee, and submit final application to register form and other documents.

Degree from one of 16 UK schools of pharmacy **or** EU equivalent **or** pass in overseas pharmacists exam

📄 Have attained the age of 21 years. **Copy of Birth Certificate***

📄 Prove your identity. **Copy of Birth Certificate***

The prerequisites to registration as a pharmacist

📄 Be in good physical and mental health. **Health declaration**

📄 Copy of degree certificate*

Pass registration exam (70% overall, including 70% on calculations section)

📄 Pay registration fee of £141 (2002) to RPSGB

📄 Complete application to register and affirmation, plus final declaration by tutor

All these documents represent the evidence that the requirement is met, and are to be supplied to RPSGB with application to register form

Figure 1.1 Registration at a glance!

1.3   Common preregistration queries: trainees

My tutor and I realise the importance of planning our workload prior to the assessments, but where do we start?

Before the actual meeting when you both discuss how you are getting on. The ideal is to meet regularly, preferably with a set agenda and realistic targets that you want to achieve; don't forget to carry out Activity M[2] to prepare you for the three RPSGB progress reports. These meetings should take place on a regular basis, and will be a formative process whereby you will be able to act on the suggestions your tutor gives you in preparation for the formal RPSGB progress review and report[3] that has to be completed at 13, 26 and 39 weeks. At these important times in your year, the appropriate forms will be completed and signed by you both. Hopefully, you will have had an induction period which introduced you to the company and its systems, and also gave you the opportunity to set targets for the year, as well as completing the initial activities referred to earlier. At the end of the meeting or formal progress review, you need to make an action plan of what to aim for next, and arrange where and when you will next review your progress, and what you need to achieve and record in the meantime. Just in case you think you have a lot to do, and that you are not getting enough guidance, go back to the original statements and your learning contract – the responsibility really is yours! However if you are unsure what to expect, or not satisfied with any aspects the process, the first person who can help is your tutor – of course it is up to you to ask, but choose the time and the place carefully.

One very important comment from an experienced tutor about the review process and the comments that are made to you. It might seem, especially at first, that you seem to be doing everything wrong and it's very easy to take all the comments the wrong way! Don't forget that the comments are constructive criticisms and meant to be formative in helping you to develop the necessary skills. Perhaps, just perhaps, that you left university with a good degree and haven't quite adapted to the very different culture where you are now expected to go back to the beginning of the learning process in some respects. It's also possible that your tutor has forgotten that you are a new trainee, not the person who was almost a pharmacist they were working with a few weeks ago. Again, the best solution is to demonstrate your maturity and ask – and reach some action points as a result.

Although it is unlikely that you will agree on every point, hopefully a working relationship will develop that encompasses individual opinions but still achieves the overall aim – that of you proving that you are competent to practice as a pharmacist.

What are my conditions of employment?

Some trainees unfortunately experience problems associated with their conditions of employment and seem to think that the Society has some sort of control over employers and their contract of employment. Whilst the *Byelaws* state the expectations of the Society, it has no powers to intervene in such matters; the general advice is to pre-empt the very rare occasions on which trouble does occur and get everything put in an official contract of employment. In the unlikely event of any problems, you will have to practice your assertiveness skills (see Section 1.8 below), or pursue a breach of the Health and Safety at Work Act.

I don't think that working in this particular pharmacy sector is for me/I am not happy with my training/my tutor – is it possible to move now? Will the time I've already completed be counted towards the 52-week total and how will it affect my entry to the next examination?

This is a tricky dilemma, and one that should be considered carefully. It is possible to complete training in two different establishments, provided that the two six-month periods are within three years (*Byelaw 19*). Even if it is possible to find another period of employment at short notice, is it necessarily going to be any better? Are the factors which you perceive to be causing the problems not, just possibly, partially your responsibility? You will also lose time when getting to know the staff and, of course, your tutor, as well as adapting to new business systems. As long as the complex administrative details and the 39-week appraisal have been completed satisfactorily, there is no reason why your examination should be delayed – but you will have to work extra hard to make up the time lost. Perhaps it might be better to persevere for the remaining time and ensure that you learn from the experience. To have identified problems and changed in order to try and overcome adverse circumstances is an example of personal qualities that other potential employers will be interested in, so long as they are presented objectively.

I have not received/I have lost my training record or receipt – how can I get another?

This question refers to the computer-generated record that each trainee receives in September, with the receipt for his or her fee. It is needed when the contractor claims their fee for being a tutor from the Health Authority, so it is not a good idea to lose it! Try sending a stamped addressed envelope with a written request for a duplicate to the Education Division.

> *What is my trainee number? I would like to have my Journal sent to a new address. Will you change the address you have on record for me?*

The two questions are posed together because the answer to them both is identical – look on the wrapper of your Journal.

> *Can I undertake preregistration training overseas?*

Initial reaction may well be 'no chance' – but you would be wrong. Under *Byelaw 18A*, up to 13 weeks can be undertaken in a pharmacy establishment within the EU; certain conditions apply, but the possibility is there.

> *Can I undertake preregistration training on a part-time basis?*

No – as stated in *Byelaw 13*, the training period should be full-time employment, for at least 52 weeks. Incidentally, the tutor also has to be a full-time employee.

1.4 Common preregistration queries: tutors

> *Does my trainee have to undertake a project during the year?*

Whilst there is definite guidance as to the knowledge, skills and behaviours that need to be acquired and/or developed, there is no absolute directive as to which learning and teaching methods should be used to reach the required standards. Whilst it might be appropriate to consider a 'project' as an alternative learning method, the advantages must be weighed carefully against the time it is likely to take, and the quantity of material that has to be covered. Another point to bear in mind, certainly for the type of in-depth study that could be expected to provide experience of research methods or a literature review, is the increased emphasis placed on the project in the revised undergraduate syllabus. Perhaps the most vital point to note is the requirement not only for the trainee to understand the fundamentals of the audit process (exam syllabus 1.1.d), but also to carry out a small, planned audit as a requirement to meet performance standard A4[4].

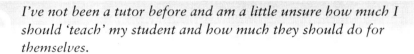

I've not been a tutor before and am a little unsure how much I should 'teach' my student and how much they should do for themselves.

A problem for many tutors, especially when confronted with a trainee who is used to/wants to be 'spoon-fed' with information. As I'm sure you appreciate, one of the main aims of the year – emphasised in the overview of the development process – is for you to 'facilitate' the learning process. The learning contract signed by the trainee, the registration exam and the whole purpose of the training year also reiterate that it is often the skills necessary to practise effectively and independently that need the most development – and you will have plenty of those. Please don't be led into thinking that you have to know everything and tell the trainee, however much easier that might be, especially at first. The tutor's Workbook[2] gives some guidance and useful case histories of strategies to be used in the event of difficulties arising in the tutoring and coaching process; there are also several activities to help with your role as a facilitator in the learning cycle.

My trainee has been off sick for X weeks. Will s/he have to extend her/his training and will her/his entry to the examination be affected?

If 'X' is more than one week, then it is a possibility. You need to contact the Education Division, who will inform the Registrar (see *Byelaw 13*), and decide each case on its individual circumstances.

My trainee is pregnant and likely to be off for X weeks. Will she have to extend her training and will her entry to the examination be affected?

As the absence is likely to be for several weeks or even months, *Byelaw 13* will again apply. The period of training can be undertaken in two parts, so long as the second starts within three years of the finish of the first (see *Byelaw 19*). Of course, there are additional difficulties caused by the end of one preregistration year and the start of the next, when the tutor may have another graduate starting. See *Byelaw 6* to clarify the position regarding the presence of more than one preregistration trainee at any time – a maximum period of 13 weeks applies.

I have been registered as a pharmacist for X years (where X is less than three). Can I be a preregistration tutor?

In normal circumstances – no (see *Byelaw 7*). An exception may be made if you take over as a preregistration tutor in the middle of a trainee's year (see *Byelaw 10*), but you would still need to have three years' pharmacy experience if you wanted to undertake the tutor's role the following year.

I have just moved into community practice from hospital. Can I be a preregistration tutor?

Sorry – no (see *Byelaw 7*).

I will be on holiday when my trainee's 13/26-week appraisal is due. Is it OK to be a couple of weeks late or should it be done early?

The guidance given by the Education Division indicates that if the appraisal is likely to be delayed for more than two weeks, then the Education Division should be informed. In fairness to all concerned it is probably better to do it a little early.

I will be on holiday when my trainee's 39-week appraisal is due. Is it OK to be a couple of weeks late or should we do it early?

The timing of the 39-week appraisal is vital; if it is late the evidence of intention to sit the examination will also be delayed, and could lead to the preregistration trainee not being eligible, or having to pay a late entrance fee.

1.5   Evidence

The following questions are mainly concerned with the initial concepts of what evidence is and why it is collected, which many students (and some tutors) do not fully understand. A much more detailed treatment of collecting evidence as part of the development process is included in the Workbook[2] and this should be referred to once the basics are understood.

Why do I have to collect evidence?

A conventional written exam is designed to test your ability to convey to the examiners a theoretical knowledge of a subject. The examiners accept your anonymous written answers as proof, or 'evidence' that you are competent – you have communicated sufficient knowledge to them to 'pass' the exam. When it comes to the assessment of practical skills and professional behaviours, it is possible to set up tutor assessed tests, but the situation does not always reflect what happens in practice. A system to meet such criteria would be extremely difficult to organise – not to say expensive. The approach now used in many workplace assessments is for trainees to present objective 'evidence' of tasks performed in the workplace to the employer or organisation responsible for maintaining standards. However, instead of a certain 'pass mark' being the indicator of success, the performance standards are used to describe 'competence' for the three key professional areas[5]. In order to help you and your tutor decide whether or not you reach the standard, behavioural indicators describe exactly what you need to do. Within the new definition of competence, it is recognised that, in addition to developing skills, the knowledge that you must have to be able to perform appropriately is an integral part; a third component of competence is the attitude needed to seek out information and create other learning activities[4]. For example, you cannot be a competent pharmacist until you meet the performance standard A2.2 – but you can't do that without a detailed knowledge of the law and the *Code of Ethics* – and the appropriate professional attitude to the need for a code[4]. The knowledge of law and ethics can also of course be tested in the registration exam.

So, how do you get to prove you are competent – well not all at once, that's for sure. Many graduates will have had experience of working in a pharmacy during vacations and may well meet some of the behavioural indicators at the beginning of the year. The activities A, B, C in the Workbook [2] are included precisely so that previous experience can be recognised and time devoted to other development needs. Don't forget that the development objectives you agree on should be SMART (Specific, Measurable, Attainable, Realistic, Timely) and reviewed regularly so that at each of the main assessments[3] you will be able to provide evidence to demonstrate competence against several behavioural indicators[5].

Is this anything to do with 'evidence-based practice' I have heard so much about?

Put very simply – yes. The onus is on you to provide objective evidence on which your tutor can ultimately make his/her judgement of your competence, rather than relying on what may be a subjective opinion. The situation is similar to that of a clinical pharmacist using the 'best' evidence (that from a primary source and based on a double-blind randomised clinical trial) to justify the inclusion of a new drug in a formulary.

What is evidence?

Many trainees (and some tutors) have difficulty in deciding what can be used as evidence. Any activity that you are asked to perform during the course of a working day could be suitable – it does not have to be (although it can be) specially organised. There's a lot more detail in your Workbook, but a simple example of an activity that could be used as evidence to comply with some criteria early on in your year is as follows:

> You take in a prescription for a prescription-only medicine (POM); the item could be for a child, but you realise that there is no age printed on the form. You check whether the patient

is under 12, and arrange for the age to be added to the form, as a legal requirement under the Medicines Act, if necessary.

The 'evidence' would need to include a photocopy of the original prescription, and an account of what was done and why. It could then be assigned to several performance criteria.

What turns this everyday activity into evidence is the formality of recording what you did – evaluating the learning outcome and which behavioural indicators[5] have been met on that occasion. Whilst one piece of evidence is not usually enough to demonstrate competence, it is often possible to use it to meet more than one behavioural indicator[5]. Using the example above, it would not take too many instances for you to demonstrate competence in the appropriate criteria.

How do I record what evidence I collect?

The simple answer is – systematically. An example is given in your Portfolio[2] of a format you may wish to follow; many companies also have their own preferred style. Remember that it is the outcome of the activity rather than the process that is important in this instance. Even if what you learnt was along the lines of 'if I meet the same situation again, I'll try a different approach', that is a most valuable learning outcome and one that can be used in your favour in discussions with your tutor.

A natural instinct might well be to collect and record as much evidence as possible and then to organise it carefully using a suitable filing method – probably the one recommended in the Portfolio[2]. Although this approach can work well, a better idea is to discriminate between quality and quantity of evidence from the start and discipline yourself only to select 'good' evidence from the beginning; don't forget that it can be used to fulfil more than one of the criteria. If you use the method described to list which pieces of evidence you have for each of the criteria and cross reference the actual evidence to all the behavioural indicators[5] that it could meet, you will save yourself a lot of work just before each progress review and assessment[3]. Then if you are a bit short of evidence for a particular behavioural indicator[5], you can identify (a), which it is, and (b), whether you have any 'dual purpose' examples tucked away that might be appropriate. If necessary, you can organise, with your tutor, situations that will enable you to provide evidence of any outstanding behavioural indicator[5].

How much evidence do I have to collect?

A facetious answer could well be: how long is a piece of string? It is, of course, quite understandable that the many behavioural indicators[5] and the need to provide evidence for them all is a daunting prospect; the secret is in careful organisation and planning.

The real answer is also completely dependent on so many variables, including the time of the year, the trainee, the tutor and the previous experience of both. The opportunity to demonstrate evidence of some of the behavioural indicators[5] can be more difficult to provide than for others, so make plans to ensure those are considered early on. Another important factor is not so much the quantity of evidence presented, but how well it is organised. A mass of photocopied prescriptions and other bits of paper is not going to be well received; an orderly folder with clear evidence of time spent on its organisation will also help with another vital feature of the assessment procedure – planning what you need to work on/achieve for the next meeting.

What is 'good' evidence?

This is a difficult question – and one that was raised by several pre-registration trainees in their questionnaires.

In addition to completing Activity L in the Workbook[2], a few general points might help:

- Agree what is and is not acceptable with your tutor.
- Try to be very concise when writing up your records.
- Try to use numbers and specific targets where possible/appropriate.
- Discuss with other trainees what is expected of them.
- Don't just compile a diary of events – make it a real learning log related to specific performance standards and behavioural indicators.
- Agree to differ at times.
- Ensure that your assessment summary[4], which is a cumulative report of your progress, is used constructively so that the evidence collected is suitable. It is also important to complete and send it to the RPSGB with each progress report.

1.6 The registration examination: administration

This is a topic that causes major difficulties: common queries and concerns are all answered here. For more detail about the content, style and sample questions refer to later chapters.

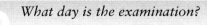
What day is the examination?

This is a vital thing to know as soon as possible if effective planning of your time is to take place throughout the year. Generally, the exam is held towards the end of June and in late September. As the date has to be notified to graduates at least six months in advance of the exam, the exact date is published in the winter bulletin; it is also in the official notices section of the Journal and in the Portfolio[2].

What books will I need to take into the examination?

Again, there is a general answer – a BNF, an MEP and a Drug Tariff. However, as in the previous question, the exact information is crucial. Each year, when the questions are written and reviewed, a particular version of each text is used. You will be at a distinct disadvantage if the book you take in is different from that used by the question setter; for example, you will not be given credit for questions that are answered incorrectly because you used the wrong book. Make sure you know exactly which books are needed from the details given in the winter bulletin. You should have no difficulty in getting a Drug Tariff, which is sent to the pharmacy every month, or the MEP, which comes directly to you with your Journal. However, if you cannot be sure that the BNF will be saved for you, it might be a good idea buy a copy. If you leave it too late, the edition you want will have been superseded; another advantage of spending about £16 in a bookshop is that you can 'customise' your copy early in preparation for the exam.

I have not received details about my examination venue or my candidate details; whom should I contact?

As this is such an important question, it is answered in several stages, ending with what do if all the other stages have been completed. Please note that if you are entering the exam other than for the first time, or are a Bradford student, or entering for the Autumn sitting, the exact timings are different; refer to your Workbook[2].

Stage 1

Check that you are eligible to sit the exam by reading the Exam Regulations. The actual entry procedure for the examination is dependent upon the following chronological events:

1   Successful completion of the 39-week progress review;
2   Submission of the completed 39-week progress report[3] together with:
3   Submission of the cumulative assessment summary[4];
4   Submission of the registration examination entry form, to be found in the Portfolio[2];
5   Payment of the examination fee, the exact amount of which can be found in the letter which is sent to all preregistration trainees, usually in late February. Make sure that you write your trainee number on the back of the cheque;
6   Submission of two passport size photos, each of which must be exactly the same and have: (i) the correct declaration on the back; and (ii) be signed by the tutor (see the Workbook[2] or the bulletin for exact details).

Stage 2

Send all the above forms to the Education Division in the envelope supplied. A checklist is printed on the back to try and reduce the number of candidates who do not send ALL the correct forms etc. at the first time of asking. No responsibility can be accepted by the Society for the late arrival of documents unless you have evidence that they were posted in good time. You are therefore strongly recommended to get a (free) certificate of posting when you send the envelope, or to send it by recorded delivery. There is no need to use registered post, as the contents have no value – except to you and your peace of mind!

It is vital that the documents reach the Society by the specified date. The exact date is notified to you in the winter bulletin, and is based on the requirement of the *Exam Regulations* to submit documents at least six weeks beforehand. You can apply up to two weeks after the closing date, but will have to pay a late entry fee (approximately double the standard fee).

Stage 3

If you have followed the procedure outlined above and have not received your letter confirming your entry and examination centre by the date specified in the bulletin, contact the exam administrators as soon as possible.

Have you received my registration exam entry?

The instructions above apply; note that you must send a stamped addressed envelope/post card if you want confirmation.

How long does the examination last and how is it structured?

No excuses for asking this question – everything is very clearly stated in the syllabus.

I am dyslexic/disabled/have a medical problem – will there be any dispensation for me?

For candidates who are ill on the day and cannot attend, the exam regulations explain very clearly what you need to do about providing evidence and transferring your attempt to the next exam. For those who have long-term problems, application must be made to the Education Division when the entrance documents are submitted. If it is felt that there were adverse circumstances on the day, again there is a strict procedure to be followed; again the details are in the exam regulations. As this is a professional exam, the general advice is that you cannot have any dispensation for such problems – there aren't any in practice.

Is there any negative marking?

Many students experience negative marking of multiple choice questions in their undergraduate days. The aim is to prevent guessing; in the Spring 1998 bulletin, a report from the examiners was summarised; the issue had been considered again, but no change is envisaged – there is no negative marking.

When will the exam results be out?

This is always a very nervous time – and the wait was extended in 1999 so that there is a gap of three weeks between sitting the exam and the notification of results. The bulletin published in May, immediately before the exam, contains exact details of when the results will be posted to you. Usually it is by first class post on Thursday evening, but, of course, there is no guarantee that they will arrive on the Friday.

How soon will I be registered after passing the examination?

Again, this will depend on several factors; if the post is on time, you should hear that you have passed on the Friday three weeks after the examination and be registered in time to start work as a pharmacist on the following Monday (that is, as long as all other requirements have been satisfied).

My tutor has not given me a satisfactory 39-week progress review – what happens now?

The situation is really serious, as you cannot sit the exam until your overall progress can be reported as being satisfactory; remedial measures need to be taken by both you and your tutor now. You will need to sit down and have an honest look at yourself and your attitude to learning. Try to be objective rather than take the easier way out and blame others. You will also need to consider whether there were any genuine extenuating circumstances that might have contributed to the failure. Then you and your tutor need to have a detailed, uninterrupted discussion covering the following points about the process and the outcomes in the hope that lost ground can be redeemed:

- Have you both read the relevant sections on progress reviews and assessments carefully, and carried out the activities if appropriate?
- Do you both fully understand the intention of the review process to be formative (to help with your development by providing milestones, feedback, guidance and monitoring) as well as summative (to assess you)?
- Do you honestly think you both tried to meet your responsibilities towards making the process succeed? Examples are planning and preparation, creating the right atmosphere for constructive discussion, etc.

○ Did you and your tutor discuss your progress or were you surprised at the outcome?

○ Were there signs in earlier appraisals that you were not developing competence as expected?

○ Were you given adequate notice, in the form of written comments, at earlier assessments and/or progress reviews and in the cumulative summaries that your progress was not meeting expectations?

○ Was there a tendency for the entries to reflect a further need to work on the more basic behavioural indicators[5] rather than demonstrating progression throughout the year?

○ Did you try to discuss any difficulties that arose in a responsible manner as they happened?

○ Did you take the advice that was offered?

○ Do you still really feel an injustice has been perpetrated?

The course of action you and your tutor decide upon will obviously depend on the exact reasons for, and the nature of, the failure. Hopefully, the discussion will have been sufficiently constructive to enable a detailed 'action plan' to be decided upon. You have to ensure that you will meet the behavioural indicator[5] and so demonstrate full professional competence in order to be able to submit a satisfactory 39-week appraisal in due course. If you work for a large company, it is likely that others will be involved in order for you to reach the desired standard. It may be that you have not had sufficient chances to demonstrate the necessary skills and behaviours, in which case your tutor will be supported in actively providing situations in which you have the necessary opportunities. If the problem is of a more fundamental nature it is probable that the Education Division at the RPSGB will be involved in a supportive, not disciplinary, role.

Another possibility is an extension to the period of preregistration training, possibly with another tutor, in order for the necessary performance criteria to be demonstrated consistently.

1.7   **Registration**

Questions from tutors

I do not think my trainee is ready for registration even though s/he has passed the examination – what should I do?

The course of action to be taken will depend on whether or not the final progress review and declaration form have been completed; if so, the preregistration trainee has fulfilled the core criteria and can register. However, if the final behavioural indicators[5] are still outstanding, and there is definite evidence that the preregistration trainee has not progressed satisfactorily from the 39-week progress review, the tutor can refuse to pass her/him on the final appraisal. In such a serious case there would have to be a very good reason, supported by evidence, which would need to be discussed with the RPSGB as a matter of urgency.

I will be on holiday for the last few weeks of my trainee's training – can somebody else sign the declaration form?

No – the 'official' tutor must sign the final declaration, although another pharmacist can help the trainee with the rest of the documents that are needed. Have another look at Fig. 1.1 to remind you both of all the pieces of paper that have to be sent to the RPSGB.

Questions from trainees

Where is my application for registration form?

Your Portfolio[2] lists the entire set of forms that need to be completed in order for registration to take place; the actual form for registration is just one of them – but it is not there. It is sent to you after your tutor has submitted evidence of your having satisfactorily completed the 39-week appraisal. If you have not received it by the date stated for your sitting of the exam contact the Education Division.

I do not have a birth certificate – will my passport be OK?

Your passport will not be sufficient on its own. You will have to complete the appropriate section of the statutory declaration (a copy is in the Portfolio[2]) which has to be done in the presence of a solicitor. Take your passport and other documents to the appointment to prove your identity – and be prepared to pay for the service s/he provides!

I have never been issued with a birth certificate but do have British nationality/identity card – is that OK?

So long as you can prove that you are the person who has gained an appropriate degree and completed the preregistration year, as well as fulfilling the other criteria, yes – as long as you follow the procedure already described for completing a statutory declaration.

I am divorced. Can I be registered in my maiden name?

Yes. If you provide your birth certificate with your registration documents you will be registered under that name. Married applicants wishing to register under their married name would need to supply their marriage certificate instead.

I have lost my degree certificate – what must I do?

You will need to contact the registration department of the university which awarded the degree as soon as possible and ask them to provide the evidence of your qualification. They will undoubtedly ask you for details such as the years during which you studied, and which course. You could also be asked for proof of identity. It may take a little while for a duplicate/copy to be issued, and again there may well be a fee.

Help – I've just seen that I have to send an affirmation – do I have to go to the solicitor and do a statutory declaration?

The 'affirmation' is a new requirement and further guidance will be provided with the application to register form. The necessity for you to complete such an undertaking is a reflection of the increased need of the body that is responsible for the regulation of pharmacists to be accountable for the quality of the individuals it admits to the register. The affirmation will be a formal document that emphasises the professional responsibilities and accountabilities that you, as a pharmacist, will be governed by, in line with other health professionals. At present the RPSGB, as the body that regulates the profession of pharmacy, sets its own guidelines for registration and regulation, although current proposals for all health professionals may lead to changes. One that is imminent is the need for mandatory continuing professional development (CPD) in order to keep up to date with changes in clinical care and practice.

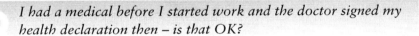

I had a medical before I started work and the doctor signed my health declaration then – is that OK?

Only if it took place immediately before starting – it must have taken place a maximum of 18 months before registration. Some companies arrange for medicals for all potential employees which take place outside the 18-month limit. In all these instances, a further examination will need to be arranged prior to registration. It can usually be done by your GP, who will then complete the health declaration in your portfolio[2]. Many doctors will need notice of the request and arrange a special appointment for which they are entitled to charge a reasonable fee.

I have not been to two branch meetings – will that hold up my registration?

The local branch is your introduction to the structure and local membership of the Society, and you are expected to be involved in its activities, and to write up the procedure as evidence to meet one or more behavioural indicators[5]. Although attendance is not an absolute requirement for registration, it is a missed opportunity for both the tutor and trainee to extend the professional relationship beyond the workplace.

Have I been registered yet?

This is the question that everyone needs to have answered before they can start work as a pharmacist – and which can only be answered by the letter from the RPSGB containing your registration number. Whilst every effort is made to send the letters out with the examination results, or immediately after they have been published, the Society is still at the mercy of the postal system. The Society has recognised that the procedure has caused problems in the past, identified the main contributory factor and consequently extended the time between the exam and the notification of results. There are several things you can do to ensure that you have the best possible chance of receiving your precious letter in time. Ensure that all the documentation regarding your registration is sent to the Society in good time, i.e. 49–50 weeks into your preregistration training. As you will no doubt have your mind on other things (i.e. the registration exam) it is a good idea to prepare as much as you can even earlier. The checklist of registration procedures that follows (see also Fig. 1.1) should help:

○ Arrange your medical to enable the health declaration to be signed sooner rather than later – and a statutory declaration if needed.
○ Get your final degree certificate and birth certificate photocopied (except for those students doing a sandwich degree).
○ Complete the 'affirmation'.
○ Fill in the application for registration form sent to you after the 39-week progress review and get your tutor to sign it.
○ Write a cheque for the amount notified to you with the application for registration form.
○ Buy, complete and stamp a postcard addressed to yourself which the Society will return to confirm that your documents have been received safely.
○ Complete the final activities that ask you to reflect on your

development throughout the preregistration training year, and to feedback to your tutor an assessment of their competency. Not only will that be a challenge in terms of the interpersonal skills that are needed, and a reversal of the whole year, it will also prepare you for some of the essential activities for when you are qualified. One is the need for an ongoing audit of your professional practice (and of course the associated CPD needs that you will identify as a result), but it will give you some practice in the sort of activity that will have to become an everyday occurrence when dealing with staff.

○ Find something else to do to take your mind off the forthcoming results – how about a well-earned break, assuming that your 52 weeks have been completed?

○ If, in spite of all possible precautions, you have not received your letter, you can ring the RPSGB after the first post on the Monday morning after publication of the results.

1.8 More complex problems

Trainees in many different types of establishments raised the following problems. Just as there is no one cause for the difficulties raised, there is certainly no one easy answer. In many of the situations described, there is, however, a common 'skill' that is perhaps not dealt with as fully as needed by many preregistration trainees in the behavioural criteria[5]. A degree of assertiveness is often necessary, which students understandably find difficult to demonstrate, especially at the beginning of the training year. Some activities are described below which are designed to enable you to become more assertive, in order to help you overcome possible problems in a constructive way. Before starting, consider the following scenarios: are these the sort of situations that you have met and do not know how to deal with?

● I am not getting the training time each week that I was promised.

- I am being treated as a pair of hands, not as a graduate.
- My tutor keeps cancelling meetings.
- My tutor has left this branch and the company has not appointed a new manager so we are having a succession of locums. Can the Society do anything?
- I'm having problems with my tutor: s/he is always critical of me and putting me down in front of other staff – what can I do?

If you can identify with the above examples, read on to find out what is meant by 'assertiveness' and for some brief ideas of how you can use the behaviour to your advantage. Remember that the recommendation from the Society is always to talk to your tutor first.

1.8.1 Some general questions about assertiveness

What is assertiveness?

Assertive behaviour allows you to express your needs, thoughts and feelings without disregarding the rights of others. It allows you to give the impression that you respect the opinion of others, but that you also have self-respect. It encourages open and honest relationships when negotiating with the many people you encounter in your working life. You will then be in a better position to influence others to provide what it is you have identified that you need.

Some more general examples of situations where assertive behaviour is appropriate are:

- Dealing with cross or aggressive customers.
- Asking for a pay rise.
- Asking someone of a higher status than you to do something which will take them some time.
- Telephoning a stranger to find out some information that you need.

Some relevant points that emerge:

- There are two aspects to assertive behaviour: whether you are the subordinate or 'boss' and whether you are asking for yourself or for others.
- Most people have most difficulty being assertive when asking for something for themselves.
- One of the great advantages of learning to behave assertively is that you begin to rate your performance independently of the response of the other person – an essential skill in many aspects of your future working life.

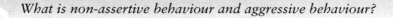

What is non-assertive behaviour and aggressive behaviour?

Many people, especially when they are in a subordinate position, demonstrate non-assertive behaviour at work, even if it is not their normal style. They act passively and allow others to dominate them; resentment builds up and wears down their confidence and self-esteem. As a further consequence, the behaviour of the person in charge becomes aggressive rather than assertive; their behaviour is often excessive and unpredictable. It communicates a message of superiority and disrespect, containing their own wants, needs and rights above those of their subordinates.

It is obvious, from the very brief description above, that such behaviour is detrimental to the working relationship and to the individuals involved.

How can I become more assertive?

1. Improve self-presentation

This is not just about wearing the right clothes and appropriate jewellery, for example, but more to do with increasing your control of the impression you make on other people. Initial impressions, as many of you will recognise, are extremely important. In addition, trying to reverse a first impression also creates problems. The very act of trying to change things might well alter someone's impression of you from that of an honest person to one where you are devious and untrustworthy.

As you enter a conversation, you not only give a visual impression, but also project an image that is used as the basis for future interactions. If the projected definition is not acceptable, further relationships will be jeopardised. Even if a favourable first impression was given, it then has to be sustained. The following influences can easily undermine self-presentation and prevent you from making and/or sustaining a favourable impression:

- If your mind wanders and your attention slips, your preoccupation will affect the image you are trying to create.
- Self-consciousness is also detrimental to your image, especially if you are trying to create an impression of interest and concern.
- If the other person is perceived to be (or is) of a much higher status within the organisation, any interaction with them can be affected due to the increased awareness of them, which undermines the impression you want to make.

All these factors demonstrate how important it is to remain in control – which requires skill and self-discipline to suppress emotional responses such as talking too much to overcome embarrassing silences.

2. Work on body language

Generally, people tend to credit themselves with much higher levels of control over the impression they make on others than is actually the case. For example, they do not realise that sitting in their usual posture, slumped in a chair with their arms folded, conveys an impression of boredom and defensiveness. In other words, impressions are made not only by how you look, but also by non-verbal signals, and, to a much lesser extent, by what you actually say! Even the tone of voice is vital; research has shown that when there is a conflict between non-verbal behaviour and what is actually said, the former wins.

Having seen very briefly the importance attached to creating the right impression, the next section goes on to consider some activities that you can use to improve your assertive behaviour.

How can I practise assertiveness?

Many people do not naturally act in a non-assertive way, but in certain situations, particularly those that are perceived as difficult or threatening, such behaviour becomes second nature. The activities below therefore concentrate on helping you to extend normal assertive behaviour to work situations.

1. Think carefully about non-verbal behaviour

- Use a firm steady voice.
- Do not blame or accuse.
- Do not threaten.
- Steady your voice when you start speaking, by saying w. . .e. . .l. . .l.
- Alternate easy phrases with ones that are difficult.

2. Change aggression to assertiveness

Try turning the following aggressive phrases that you might have heard/made in the workplace to assertive ones, by changing them from a 'you' to an 'I' statement in four stages:

- Begin with 'I'.
- Describe what you think, feel or need.
- Describe the other person's behaviour that led to your need.
- Describe what changes you want and why you need them.

Try with these examples:

- You always tell me to stop what I am doing and answer the telephone.
- You have made another mistake in the CD register.
- You always give me another job to do before I have finished the last one.

Some further hints:

- Use factual descriptions rather than judgements.
- Showing needs and feelings means you are less likely to put the recipient on the defensive and provoke aggressive responses.
- Express thoughts and feelings to show your involvement.
- Use direct requests like 'I think it would be a good idea if you . . .'
- Show that you have listened by acknowledging their contribution.
- Try repeating yourself if the expressed need is not met the first time round. The method is called the 'broken record' and means that if you continue on the same theme without distraction, you will eventually force them to listen to you. Be careful, as the use of force or coercion may lead to the breakdown of the relationship. Show that you are also empathetic to the other person.
- If you are not sure as to why someone is behaving in a particular way – ask. Remember to be very careful to keep your tone

of voice assertive rather than aggressive so as not to appear blaming.

○ If you thought that an agreement had been reached, but it is not being implemented, a question must be asked which draws attention to the situation without being rude or aggressive. An example would be: 'I thought that after the last appraisal I was going to get more practice in taking in prescriptions; I'm still very keen to do that.'

○ If you have a sanction available to you, use it as a last resort; for example, to get action when every other approach has been unsuccessful. Remind the person concerned of the consequences of their behaviour to themselves. Be very careful, as it can so easily be interpreted as aggression – but if you have a lot to lose if a change is not forthcoming, it may be your only option. Wait until they must realise that your patience has been tried too far, and that you really need to impress on them that you are serious.

Now, try using the points outlined on a situation which you have had difficulty with, but is not the most vital issue you want to tackle.

Afterwards, reflect on the level of assertiveness you demonstrated by scoring each of the following numbered points on a scale from 1 (non-assertive) to 5 (aggressive), which are described in Table 1.2.

If your total score was high (e.g. more than 22), or low (less than 10), some of your behaviour would have been interpreted as aggressive or non-assertive, respectively. Try to identify which aspects of your behaviour you need to work on and practice again before using what you have learnt on really important issues.

1.9   Summary

1.9.1   What's hot and what's not

The following lists are a very brief summary of some of the features of the new programme and those that are no longer felt to be

Table 1.2   An assertiveness scale

| | 1........................3...........................5 | | | 'Score' |
	Non-assertive	Assertive	Aggressive	
1. Verbal content	Few 'I' statements	Clear, unemotional description of the facts	Unnecessary 'I' statements	
	Fill in words		Opinions made facts	
	Apologies	Constructive criticism without blame or assumptions	Advice with lots of 'oughts' and 'shoulds'	
	Frequent justifications			
		Questioning of the thoughts and needs of others	Use of sarcasm	
			Exaggerates	
2. Tone of voice	Anxious	Confident	Sarcastic	
	Nervous laughter	Assured	Arrogant	
	Apologetic	Warm	Very firm	
	Soft	Sincere	Condescending	
3. Facial expression	Waiting for rebuke	Open-smiles when pleased, frowns when angry	Tight jaw	
	Pleading		Tense	
		Relaxed mouth	Tight lips	
	Quick changing features	Few blinks	Frowning	
			Threatening	
4. Eye contact	Evasive	Firm without staring	Stares	
5. Body posture	Wants to appear insignificant	Erect	Taut and rigid	
6. Body movements	Wringing hands	Head held high with nodding	Finger pointing	
	Shuffles feet		Clenched hands	
	Shrugs	Open hand movements	Walks around impatiently	

appropriate. They are not intended to be comprehensive, but to give a few concluding thoughts as to how the preregistration training programme has developed.

What's hot

- Use of email and the Internet.
- Direct dial phone numbers to the appropriate section at the education department of the RPSGB.
- A patient-orientated programme to reflect changes in the NHS.
- Recognition of the differing needs of tutors and the opportunity to develop skills as individual CPD.
- Cross-sector experience to enable new skills to be developed.
- More emphasis on calculations without a calculator in the exam.
- More empathy to the needs of trainees in the revised layout and content of resources.
- Recognition that pharmacists from overseas and sandwich students undertake the programme in a different way.
- Recognition of the importance of self-assessment of skills etc. for both the trainee and the tutor.
- A structured set of activities to develop vital skills.
- Emphasis on the need for knowledge, skills and attitudes to be integrated in the performance standards – but a daunting list of 'extra' knowledge requirements.
- Completely revised syllabus to reflect major changes in practice and the NHS.
- Responsibility for learning placed firmly on the trainee with the contract.
- Personal responsibility for providing appropriate support with the 'agreement to tutor,' the byelaws and the changes to the *Code of Ethics*.
- Forms which are clearly labelled with the RPSGB crest.
- More diagrams to illustrate concepts such as the learning cycle.

- More clarification of what is needed as evidence.
- Problem-based approach to the registration exam supported by the emphasis on questions that demand analysis and evaluation rather than recall of knowledge.
- A revised *Code of Ethics* with specific reference to the demands of acting as a preregistration tutor.
- Assessments and summaries of progress.
- Developing from a (sub)consciously incompetent trainee to a consciously competent newly registered pharmacist.
- SMART objectives.
- The use of a 'learning log'.
- Submission of all forms and documents to the RPSGB on time and in the proscribed format.
- The challenge of the registration exam.
- The satisfaction of successfully meeting the challenges and registering as a pharmacist.

What's not so hot/on the way out

- An exam syllabus that contained many topics already covered at undergraduate level.
- Definitive list of texts to be kept at each shop with a pre-registration trainee.
- Competence measured as a consistent performance of sector-specific skills.
- A huge manual with masses of information and vital forms which is difficult to access.
- Compulsory attendance at the RPSGB for dissemination of information to all new tutors, regardless of their previous experience.
- Self-reliance on the identification of suitable development exercises to be recorded as evidence.
- Appraisals.
- Administration of the exam by Edexcel.

1.9.2 Summary of alternative references for CBTP users

The following references are referred to by a superscript number in the text:

1 Competence Based Training Programme.
2 Manual/manual section for tutors.
3 Appraisal and/or report.
4 There is no equivalent requirement in the CBTP.
5 In the CBTP, the equivalent to the three key professional areas and performance standards (described by behavioural indicators) are the four professional elements and the three practical units which are qualified by very detailed 'performance criteria' and by definitions for guidance. The definition of competence is 'having the necessary skills, knowledge and attitudes to undertake the role of a pharmacist properly and consistently'. However, the associated knowledge is not always part of the criteria against which the preregistration trainee is measured. That means that, on occasions, the knowledge to underpin practice has to be checked separately as it cannot be assumed within the observed behaviour. Such knowledge is indicated by an 'I' whereas the activities that should be undertaken are indicated by an 'E'.
6 Performance criteria.

The terminology to be used to enable those following the Competence Based Training Programme to find the appropriate resource is shown in Table 1.3.

Table 1.3

	Terminology used in the CBTP	Terminology used in the TPAP
Terminology associated with assessment of training	1. Progress review 2. Appraisal report 3. None	Progress review Progress report Assessment summary

2

Calculations without a calculator

2.1 The rationale for not allowing calculators in the preregistration examination

The exam syllabus, regulations and recent articles have made very clear the position of the Boards of Examiners regarding the requirement for preregistration trainees to be able to perform calculations without a calculator. A brief explanation of the Society's views are given in the exam guidance notes, and there is also further evidence of the correlation between the ability to perform calculations under duress without a calculator and failure. In a recent exam almost half the trainees who failed scored less than 50% on the calculation questions. The new syllabus is even more explicit with regard to the ability to be able to perform simple calculations without a calculator. There are now 20 calculation-style questions in a separate section on the open book paper, with a pass mark of 70%. Instead of reading the chapter any further, pause for the time allowed for one open-book question (just under two minutes) and try to work out, *without a calculator,* how many calculation questions can be wrong before a pass becomes a failure.

The number to get wrong and still pass is 6, which is probably a far easier question than the vast majority that will be encountered. For many, that will be a daunting number, and of course it's not a good idea to cut it too fine and rely on only getting a few wrong. The aim for the diagnostic questions (to be completed at the start of the year as a vital self assessment of current competence towards the need for 'development' in this area of the syllabus) is for a 'pass mark' of 80%. Any difficulties identified as a result can then be worked on before it's too late. Tutors are advised that they should not sign the 39-week appraisal for tutees who don't by then achieve 70% – which means that they cannot be entered for the registration exam unless and until they can demonstrate competence. Although the position is reviewed every year, it is unlikely to change in the immediate future. Perhaps a first step for those who are 'concerned' (read paranoid) is to make a resolution to study the rest of the chapter now – it might just provide the key to answering some of your problems.

The RPSGB Council quite rightly insists that those admitted to the register of pharmaceutical chemists must be able to perform calculations accurately. Preregistration trainees are equally convinced about the need to be accurate; it is the requirement to be able to do the calculations without the use of a calculator in the examination that they question.

The demand is based on the premise that calculators are used without a basic understanding of the underlying numbers; consequently, arithmetical mistakes are made, with potentially fatal results. The current concern of the RPSGB (and others) is encompassed in the concept of what used to be called a 'sense of number' – and the fact that it appears to be lacking in many of today's graduates. The cause, and the exact definition, is not at issue; what is important is the concept and what it means in practice. Banning the use of calculators means that graduates have to use their arithmetical skills, which involve a 'sense of number' – and by doing so, reduce the possibility of making potentially fatal arithmetical errors. The process is summarised in Fig. 2.1.

2.2 Understanding why a 'sense of number' is essential for practice

Having established that a 'sense of number' is vital to success, it is appropriate to consider the exact meaning in this context. As with the rest of this chapter, examples from practice and from sample examination papers will be used to demonstrate the relevance of the concept before going on to consider how the necessary skills can be developed – rapidly.

A consideration of the following points can demonstrate the value of the procedure:

Figure 2.1   A summary of the rationale for the absence of calculators.

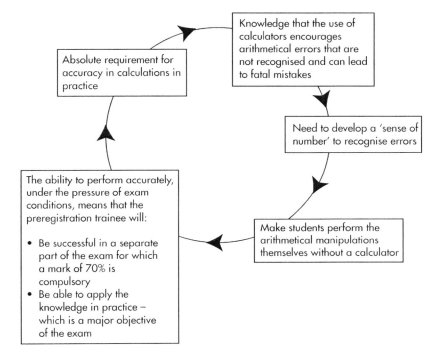

In the days before calculators were invented (your parents will
remember them well), it was common practice to look at the
'sum' and roughly estimate the magnitude of the answer.
From that relatively simple procedure (at least it is when you
always do it as a matter of habit), some vital, practice-related
outcomes can result.

A mistake in substituting values – for example the use of mg
instead of mcg – can be quickly spotted.

It prevents long, tortuous manipulations of the wrong
numbers.

If an arithmetical mistake is subsequently made, it can be
quickly spotted and the calculation checked.

In other words, having an expected order of value with which to compare the answer should prevent an arithmetical error – that anyone can make under pressure – actually being administered as a dose. In the present context, the 'sense of number' means even more: it also includes the ability to spot quickly connections between numbers and to have a sense of when the answer must be smaller or larger than the original quantity.

The converse situation happens with a calculator: the sum is put in wrongly, or the wrong button pressed, and because the calculator (but not the operator) is infallible, the answer is taken as true and written down without a second glance. At no stage is there any attempt to ask the question 'does it make sense?' Even when – or if – that question is posed, either by tutors or by the graduates themselves, the ability to stand back and look at the problem again objectively is also lacking.

Another even more worrying technique arises with students who do not understand the concepts; they try the sum with the figures in every possible combination until a plausible (to them) answer appears. You will find that the incorrect answers in multiple choice questions always include those that arise from having the numbers wrongly arranged – particularly with scaling up and down calculations. The question setters, examiners and Council members are wise to such practices and seek to prevent the students who do not understand the concepts from registering as pharmacists – by insisting that no calculators can be used in the registration exam.

An example will hopefully convince you of the theory:

How much potassium permanganate would be needed to prepare one litre of a 1 in 2000 solution?

A ☐ 200 mg   B ☐ 500 mg   C ☐ 1 g   D ☐ 2 g   E ☐ 5 g

The correct answer is B; the solution is 1 in 2000, which converts to 0.05%, so to make 1 litre, 0.5 g (500 mg) is needed. If the 1 in 2000 is calculated to be 0.5%, then the answer is E, and if the concept of parts misunderstood so that the percentage strength is

0.02% or 0.2%, then answers A and D, respectively, are given. Although the potassium permanganate is used externally, the principle is of much greater importance when applied to potent medications for systemic use.

2.2.1   Using a 'sense of number': some examples

So, the calculator is being removed from your grasp for a very good reason – to encourage the use of a 'sense of number'. To take the argument a little further – because there is no need to perform laborious mathematical manipulations, the temptation is to resort to the use of a calculator without thinking about the answer to the sum. If you have to think 'how on earth am I going to work that out', you may learn to think first 'what is the rough answer' and then work it out exactly. Furthermore, if your rough estimate is obviously wrong for what you might expect – for example, as a dose of a potent drug – then you have not only avoided a lot of effort for yourself, but perhaps saved the life of a very sick baby that would otherwise have been given an overdose. In other words, using a 'sense of number' gives you a rough estimate before calculating the exact answer; in the exam, you may find that you need to go no further – there is only one possible answer from the choices provided.

The following simple example can be used to illustrate how the principle can be used to your advantage:

A prescriber orders 75 g of a cream containing 2.5% of sulphur in a base of aqueous cream. How much sulphur must be weighed out?

A ☐ 3.33 g   B ☐ 2.5 g   C ☐ 2.25 g   D ☐ 1.88 g   E ☐ 1.5 g

As you know that 2.5% means 2.5 g in 100 g, the answer must be less, because the 75 g which you have to make is less than 100 g – so the response should never be A and B, whatever the calculator might have said!

The fact that 75 g is three-quarters of 100 g means that you should be able to do the sum very quickly – if you understand 'fractions' and 'cancelling' (if not, see below).

The answer is equivalent to $^3/_4$ of 2.5 g

$$= \frac{3 \times 2.5}{4} = 7.5 \div 4.$$

You may not be able to work out what that is quickly – but then you don't have to; remember that the best way to check a division sum is to take what you think the answer is/could be and multiply it by the number you were trying to divide by. However poor your knowledge of tables, you should know that $2 \times 4 = 8$, which means that it cannot be C, because $2.25 \times 4 =$ much more than 8, and you know the answer to the checking procedure must be 7.5.

So your 'sense of number' says that D or E must be the only possible answers without doing any dividing. Most will not need to guess but be able to divide exactly to get the answer 1.875, so the correct code is D.

But – using the previous argument, keep trying the multiplying rather than the much harder dividing. If the only two possible answers are D and E, it doesn't take a moment to multiply $1.5 \times 4 = 6$ – you can quickly see that it's too small.

However, $1.88 \times 4 = 7.52$ (the exact answer is actually $^3/_4$ of $2.5 = 1.875$).

Another (open-book) example where the numbers are harder, and the technique of estimating even more worthwhile, is:

The recommended dose of diclofenac for a child is 3 mg/kg/day. What is the most appropriate number of paediatric suppositories to be used daily for a 5-year-old child of average weight?

A ☐ 3   B ☐ 4   C ☐ 2   D ☐ 5   E ☐ 6

From the BNF, a child of five weighs 18 kg, so the daily dose is 3×18 mg. As each suppository contains 12.5 mg, the number required is

$$\frac{3 \times 18}{12.5}$$

There is no need to do the sum – a 'sense of number' will immediately enable you to see that 18 and 12 are linked – they both divide (cancel) by 6. The sum becomes much easier as

$$3 \times 3 \div 2 = 4.5$$

You then have the problem of deciding between answers B and D – but you should realise that it is not advisable to recommend a number of suppositories that would, in effect, give more than 3 mg/kg/day, so go for the lower number – the answer is B.

Perhaps the most worrying aspect of candidates' lack of a sense of number arises when calculations are performed involving factors of 10. A case featured in the media involved a calculation error of two decimal places, which resulted in the tragic death of a baby. The concerns of the RPSGB were reported in detail and the need to be able to handle decimal points correctly without a calculator made absolutely clear.

The emphasis in Chapter 2 is therefore to introduce or revise techniques, however basic, to help you do calculations without your calculator in the exam. If you can perform at a satisfactory level under the pressure of an exam situation, then you have every chance of being able to do it in practice – which is, after all, what the exam is designed to test.

2.3   A rationale for the lack of a 'sense of number' in pharmacy graduates

It is quite possible that many tutors (and others), especially if more 'mature' in years, will wonder what this chapter is doing in a book aimed at graduates in a scientific discipline. After all, 'they' had no problem passing the '11 plus', using a slide rule/log tables for O-levels, or even passing A-level maths before calculators were invented. Given a calculator and/or a personal computer, preregistration trainees can plot complex graphs, work out standard deviations and perform numerous other mathematical operations. However, a relatively simple sum, under exam conditions and without a calculator, causes many candidates to really struggle. One only has to observe the pages of sums covering the question papers in 'mock' exams to know that much time and effort has been wasted – perhaps to no avail.

The reasons for the situation may well be connected with the way that arithmetic was taught in primary schools in the 1980s. Whatever those reasons prove to be, it is the consequences, not the theories and how they are resolved, which is the current concern. From discussions with, and observations of, many preregistration trainees, it is apparent that there are a significant number who reluctantly admit that it is not the initial stage of substituting the numbers into the formula where they lack confidence/ability, but in knowing how to perform the basic arithmetic to solve the sum. For most preregistration trainees there is ample evidence that it is the arithmetic in the calculations where they really need help. Consider the following recent statement from a preregistration trainee as an example, if one were needed:

> . . . but if I divide 1 by 10 I get −9 and that answer isn't one of the possibilities!

Frightening but true. The actual point at which students commonly fail has been a revelation to tutors and to others; it now needs to be remedied – fast.

2.4 Techniques to enable you to develop a 'sense of number' – quickly

So swallow your pride, and admit that, probably through no fault of your own, a sense of number is what you need to master. That admission is the first step in a process that will enable you to get to grips with some of the techniques described. Remember that you don't have to confess to others that this is the level at which you have problems – although lots have, which is why it is included. Just recognise your own difficulties and take the opportunity to overcome them. There is nothing too hard – it is just learning techniques which may never have been explained to you before.

If you are one of the very few who can confidently do the necessary arithmetic and gain at least 80% in the diagnostic calculations *without* the use of a calculator, please don't be insulted that the topic is included and go straight onto the next chapter – perhaps after having done the examples.

So, having accepted, however unwillingly, the argument for not being able to use a calculator, and that you need to improve your arithmetical skills sufficiently, what can be done? And how can the techniques be learnt quickly and utilised in actual exam questions? That is what the following pages are all about. In order to identify the arithmetical techniques that are needed to answer the examination questions, two calculation papers issued by the Education Division were analysed. The results of the analysis are presented in Table 2.1.

Although in many of the questions more than one technique was necessary, it was interesting to note that nothing more complicated than knowledge of the multiplication tables up to 12 was involved. There were no examples where long division was necessary, for instance. It is hopefully comforting to note that there are only four basic skills that you need to acquire and be able to apply. Each of the identified techniques is explained briefly before some suggestions for individual practice are given. Don't forget – it doesn't matter how obvious some of the ideas are; if they can help you, then use them.

2.4.1 Arithmetical techniques: linking fractions, decimals, percentages and 'parts'

Many students recognise that a decimal is much easier to deal with than a fraction, but a surprising number cannot convert them.

Taking the first point:

Which is the largest number from the following?

☐ 6/7   ☐ 4/5   ☐ 5/6   ☐ 8/10   ☐ 7/8

It probably takes a few minutes to work out (guess?) that it's 7/8. Incidentally, did you spot that 4/5 and 8/10 are identical amounts? If the same numbers are presented as decimals: 0.8, 0.83, 0.875, 0.857, even mixed up, it is not too difficult to see that 0.875 is largest.

It is also much easier to manipulate figures expressed as decimals – so make sure you can convert them, then it's an easy step to work in percentages too. Remember, it's not the concept of percentages that is the issue here, but being able to work them out from fractions and 'parts' without the trial and error method adopted with a calculator.

To help you see the connection between fractions and decimals, remember that a fraction simply represents one number divided by another one which is bigger: i.e. $^3/_4$ really means 3 divided by 4, which is $3.0 \div 4 = 0.75$ (4 can't be divided into 3, but it can go into 30, seven times with a remainder of 2. It then goes into 20 five times. Keep the decimal point in the correct place and the conversion is complete. To change to a percentage, multiply by 100 by moving the decimal point two places to the right – 75%.)

For those who need a reminder about working with decimals, consider these examples of calculations that depend on the ability to use powers of 10.

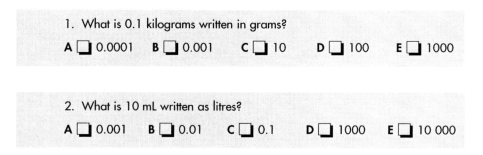

1. What is 0.1 kilograms written in grams?

A ☐ 0.0001   B ☐ 0.001   C ☐ 10   D ☐ 100   E ☐ 1000

2. What is 10 mL written as litres?

A ☐ 0.001   B ☐ 0.01   C ☐ 0.1   D ☐ 1000   E ☐ 10 000

Table 2.1 The analysis of RPSGB calculations papers November 1998 and March 1999

Paper/ question number	Arithmetical techniques used to solve each problem					
	1 Fractions/ percentages/ decimals/ parts	2 Cancelling/ dividing	3 Scaling up and down			4 Other
			(i) Doses	(ii) Formulae	(iii) Concentrations	
November 1998						
1			✓			
2		✓				
3					✓	
4			✓			
5		✓	✓			
6	✓					
7				✓		
8				✓		
9				✓		
10			✓			
11	✓				✓	
12				✓		
13	✓				✓	✓
14		✓			✓	
15	✓	✓			✓	
16	✓			✓		✓
17				✓		
18		✓		✓		
19			✓			
20				✓		
Spring 1999						
1			✓			
2	✓				✓	
3				✓		
4			✓			
5				✓		
6			✓			
7			✓			
8			✓			
9			✓			
10		✓			✓	
11				✓		
12				✓		
13				✓		
14				✓		
15		✓	✓			
16		✓	✓			
17						✓
18		✓			✓	
19			✓			
20	✓		✓			

A 'sense of number' in this context means that in question 1, a conversion from kilograms to grams, the answer must be a larger number because grams are smaller – so A and B can be instantly dismissed. You will probably know that there are 1000 g in 1 kg (and 1000 mcg in 1 mg) so E is also wrong. There are still many candidates who will multiply 0.1 by 1000 to get 10 and answer C and not the correct answer D. Similar problems arise with converting 10 mL to litres by dividing 10 by 1000 to get A instead of B.

A reminder of how to multiply and divide decimals without a calculator

To multiply a whole number by 10, 100, 1000, etc., attach as many '0's to the right of the whole number as there are in the number you are multiplying by (the multiplier).

> i.e. To multiply 345 by 100, add two '0's to give 34 500

To multiply a number with a decimal point by 10, 100, 1000, etc., move the decimal point as many places to the right as there are '0's in the multiplier. Remember to add additional '0's as needed.

> i.e. To multiply 678.91 by 1000, you need to move the point three places to the right. As there are only two figures after the decimal point, you need to add a '0' at the end first; the answer is 678 910.

To divide any number by 10, 100, 1000 etc., move the decimal point to the left as many times as there are '0's in the divisor. Remember to add some '0's if necessary before the number you are dividing.

> i.e. To divide 123.456 78 by 10 000, you need to move the decimal point four places to the left, so put another 0 in front first to give four places to move it to. It is also customary to add a 0 before the decimal point to ensure that it is not lost. The answer is 0.012 345 678, written as 0.012 345 678.

Parts

Calculations using 'parts' are not unique to pharmacy; however, others who use them – people who mix paint, for example – have a very helpful machine to do it for them. You don't, even though the end result is a lot more critical than an exact match for the curtains!

To relate them all, try Exercise 2.1, which involves filling in the blank spaces. The numbers are easy to start with and get harder, but they can all be done with a good knowledge of the multiplication tables. The answers are towards the end of the chapter in Section 2.6.

Exercise 2.1

Fraction (as the smallest number)	Part	Decimal	Percentage
Example above: 3/4	3 in 4	0.75	75
1/4		0.25	
	1 in 100		1
	. . . in 1000	0.2	
2/5			
	1 in 80		
	. . . in 10 000	0.04	
			45

Have a look at the following example, which many students could not do when presented with it in a 'mock' exam.

A pharmacist is required to send 100 mL of a solution of chlorhexidine gluconate, which when diluted 1 in 10, produces a 1 in 1000 solution. The pharmacist has available a 500 mL bottle of a solution of 20% w/v chlorhexidine gluconate. The correct formula will be:

A ☐ Chlorhexidine gluconate concentrate 1 mL, water to 100 mL
B ☐ Chlorhexidine gluconate concentrate 2 mL, water to 100 mL
C ☐ Chlorhexidine gluconate concentrate 5 mL, water to 100 mL
D ☐ Chlorhexidine gluconate concentrate 10 mL, water to 100 mL
E ☐ Chlorhexidine gluconate concentrate 20 mL, water to 100 mL

Most students will want to use the formula $C_1V_1 = C_2V_2$, where C_1 and C_2 and V_1 and V_2 refer to the initial and final concentrations and volumes respectively. For most trainees, the difficulty arises when going onto the next stage. To substitute in the formula, you need to write down which quantities you have and which you need to calculate. In order to demonstrate the points later, the phrase from the question that leads to the value is included.

> C_1 = has available a 500 mL bottle of a solution of 20% w/v
> V_1 = ?
> C_2 = when diluted 1 in 10, produces a 1 in 1000 solution
> V_2 = to send 100 mL

The problem that is most encountered is the final concentration C_2, as it is not given clearly. What is actually needed is a 1 in 100 solution, as 'when it is diluted 1 in 10 it must make a 1 in a 1000 solution', i.e. the solution provided to the customer must be 10 times stronger. Even if you can reach this stage, your problems are not over as the two concentrations are not in the same units. '1 in 100' needs to be changed to a percentage before the sum can be done – not too difficult but, unless the terminology is understood, absolutely impossible. In this instance it is recognised by most that 1 in 100 is 1%; other examples are much harder. Substitution and calculation can then be carried out:

> $C_1V_1 = C_2V_2$
>
> $20 \times ? = 1 \times 100,$
>
> so $? = \dfrac{1 \times 100}{20}$

Now comes the bit that is the real clue to working without a calculator – knowing your tables! Both 100 and 20 divide by 5 and by 4 (and of course by 20), so the answer is

> = 5 mL

(As the units of volume for V_2 are mL, the same is true of V_1.)
From the choices above, the answer is C.

2.4.2 Arithmetical techniques: 'cancelling' – or dividing quickly

This is something that those of us used to working without a calculator do almost automatically when confronted by any sum, but if you have never had to bother, it can be a real obstacle to success in the calculations. The secret, of course, is knowing one's times tables – the example above is just one where it's essential. That doesn't mean 'knowing' as in going along on your fingers saying under your breath 'seven ones are 7, 'seven twos are 14', etc., but instantly saying '56' when someone says 'seven eights', for example. There is no doubt that spending some time here will pay dividends. A quote in *The Times* (18 April 1999), describing the reasons for the introduction of the 'numeracy hour' in primary schools, put the problem succinctly:

> 'Pupils who find it difficult to learn their tables have to get to the stage at which they realise how much easier life would be if they knew them . . . if you don't know them well, it's like driving and having to think each time you change gear.'

To demonstrate the point, look at the following very simple example.

A patient with cardiovascular disease is prescribed Gaviscon Advance, 10 mL qds. The prescriber asks the pharmacist how many mmol of sodium ions the patient is taking from his medication in 24 hours. Which one of the following is correct?

A ☐ 8   B ☐ 18.4   C ☐ 24.8   D ☐ 46   E ☐ 92

By looking in the BNF you discover that Gaviscon Advance contains 2.3 mmol Na^+/5 mL. As the patient takes 40 mL a day, the total daily dose in mmol is

$$\frac{2.3 \times \overset{8}{\cancel{40}}}{\cancel{5}}$$

If you don't know your eight times table (five eights are 40), it will take you longer than it should to cancel and leave the final sum as $2.3 \times 8 = 18.4$, and mark your answer, as B. Remember, in the original exam you had 70 'open-book' questions in two hours, which is $120/70 = 1.7$ minutes each, on average – not very long when some questions are much more complex and you also have to look up at least one and sometimes two or three references in the BNF. The number of questions in the new open book paper is now 80, to be completed in 2.5 hours – which is still a testing $150/80 = 1.875$ minutes per question. However the recommended time for the 20 calculations is one hour, which is 3 minutes each, but that of course only leaves 90 minutes for 60 questions, or 1.5 minutes each.

Other general exercises to help

When dispensing, always work out the number of tablets needed in your head first – and don't let anyone tell you the answer! Courses of prednisolone and strips of 14 tablets are a good example.

Tricks for dividing

If you want to check if a large number is divisible by 3 (or 30 or 300), add up all the digits – if the resultant number is divisible by 3, then the original will be too! For example:

$$\frac{3579}{3}$$

$3 + 5 + 7 + 9 = 24$ which is divisible exactly by 3, so 3579 is too (answer = 1193).

To divide by 25, move the decimal point two places to the left (i.e. divide by 100) and then multiply by 4. For example:

$$\frac{180\ 007\ 525}{25} = 1\ 800\ 075.25 \times 4 = 7\ 200\ 301$$

Any number that is divisible by 5 ends in 0 or a 5.

2.4.3   Arithmetical techniques: scaling up and down

As with so many of the other topics in this section, the concept is a real stumbling block for students, and a prime target for those who put all the possible combinations of the numbers in the calculator. It is also taught totally differently from the formal equation based on the principle 'if you know three things, you can always calculate the fourth', which is described below. The problem is not just recognising the type of problem, but knowing which number to put where. As there are many variations on the theme of increasing and decreasing quantities, it is vital to really understand the procedure.

The foolproof formula that some have found better than the 'if you want to make it bigger, multiply by the larger number' approach is best shown in some examples.

---

350 g of an ointment containing 12.5% w/w of a single active ingredient has been prepared. The weight of active ingredient contained in 140 g of ointment is:

A ☐ 4.8 g   B ☐ 11.0 g   C ☐ 13.4 g   D ☐ 14.5 g   E ☐ 17.5 g

---

From the question, take the statement of % as the starting point, i.e. 12.5% w/w, which immediately gives you the amount in 100 g (forget the 350 g), which is the first line of the formula:

12.5 g in 100 g is equivalent to

? g in 140 g.

Then follow the same procedure every time: put the unknown ? in the top left-hand corner and keeping the statement of % as before, the ratio of ? to 12.5 equals the ratio of 140 to 100, so write the four things in that same order, i.e. as the 'foolproof formula':

$$\frac{?}{12.5} = \frac{140}{100}$$

Then turn it round to give ? on its own – and solve the sum.

So,   ? $= \dfrac{140 \times 12.5}{100}$

which is the same as:

$$\dfrac{14 \times 12.5}{10}$$

'Cancel' by dividing top and bottom by 5

$$\dfrac{14 \times \cancel{12.5}^{\,2.5}}{2\ \cancel{10}}$$

to give

$$\dfrac{14 \times 2.5}{2}$$

then cancel again by dividing by 2

$$\dfrac{\cancel{14}^{\,7} \times 2.5}{\cancel{2}_{\,1}}$$

to give 7 × 2.5 = 17.5 g or (E).

Exercise 2.2 below enables you to test yourself on the main types of arithmetical techniques already identified in Table 2.1.

The second column has a calculation in it; you do not need to use any other reference sources – all the information you need is given. The third column has the answer, and the fourth an equivalent. In the exam you have also have a choice of answers; however, this differs in that there are more than four 'distracters'.

Note that the fractions, where given, are for your practice, not because they would be presented to you like that. The units to be attached to the quantity in column 2 are shown in the question, e.g. dose/mg.

Exercise 2.2   Basic calculations test

	Question (you need to solve the sum in each case)	Answers to choose from	Equivalents to match to answer in column 3
1	Dose (in mg) in 0.2 mL of an injection containing 6 mg/mL	1	250 mg
2	Volume (in mL) that contains 5 mg if the injection is 15 mg/2 mL	1/2	3600 mg
3	Dose (in mcg) in 1/10 mL of an injection containing 450 mcg/mL	1/4	0.02 L
4	Active ingredient (in g) in 30 g of an ointment containing 12% w/w	600	0.15 g
5	Dose (in mg) of drug at 6 mg/kg for a 25 kg child	1.2	1.2 g
6	Mass of potassium permanganate (in g) in 250 mL of solution containing 1 part in 1000	1200	1/10 of 80
7	Volume (in mL) of an 8% w/v solution containing 40 mg	1600	0.045 L
8	Volume (in mL) of syrup to add so that a mixture containing 0.5 mg in 1 mL contains 2 mg/5 mL; 100 mL needed	9	0.045 mg
9	Total amount of drug (in mg) infused after two hours at 10 mg/minute	1800	1200 mcg
10	Total volume of solution (in mL) given at 10 drops/minute for 90 minutes if 1 drop is 0.05 mL	210	0.667 mL
11	% of active ingredient if a 40% solution is diluted 1 in 5	1/3 of 2	1/20 of 40 000
12	% of active ingredient if a 45% solution is diluted by taking 1 part and adding 4 parts	0.1	1.8 g
13	Volume (in mL) taken if a 15% solution is diluted to give 300 mL of 5%	7	1/4 of 6.4 g
14	Total daily dose (in mg) of a drug given to a 7 kg baby at a level of 10 mg/kg tds	2000	0.001 kg

continued overleaf

Exercise 2.2 (continued)

		Question (you need to solve the sum in each case)	Answers to choose from	Equivalents to match to answer in column 3
	15	Total daily dose (in mg) of a drug given to a 20 kg child at a level of 15 mg/kg qqh	70	1/50 of 2500
	16	Total amount of drug (in g) if 250 mg given qds for one week	100	1/200 of 1400 g
	17	Total dose of drug (in mg) at 5 mg/kg/day for 20 days to a 16 kg child	150	0.08 kg
	18	Dose (in mg) to give a 30 kg child at 20 mg/kg	3.6	100 mcg
	19	Number of mmol in 112 g of drug if the M_r = 56	50	1/9 of 5.4 g
	20	Volume (in mL) of a 0.1 Molar solution to give 5 mmol of active ingredient	45	70 000 g
	21	The weight (in kg) of an 11 stone man. 1 kg = 2.2 lb, 14 lb = 1 stone	45	0.1 L
	22	The weight of cream (in g) to use for 200 g of a preparation that is base:cream in ratio of 3:2	20	1/7 th of 1470
	23	The weight of solid (in g) to use for 200 mL of a solution such that when diluted 40 times, a 1 in 8000 solution is produced	8	1/100 of 900
	24	The amount of drug (in mg) in 0.1 mL of a 1 in 1000 solution	80	500 mcL

2.5   Sample multiple choice questions (MCQs)

The calculations that are presented below cover the range of arithmetical skills previously identified in the papers analysed. They are presented in the same four styles of MCQs as in the registration exam; details are on p. 129. A few points to note:

- The separate section of 20 calculation questions is on the open-book paper, but for both some of the questions in the exam and for these examples there is no need to consult a reference source.
- As the calculation questions are such a vital part of preparing for the exam, and a major source of worry to so many, you will have to consider carefully whether or not to try them now, or leave them for a little while – perhaps until you have read the next chapter.
- The aim of the exam questions – to test the skills of analysis and evaluation – and the implications to those concerned is covered in more detail later. However that demand, in addition to testing the basic arithmetic techniques described above, means that you might find the questions a little difficult at first and it might be better to concentrate on the exercises at first. Whenever you do decide to test yourself, do the MCQs without a calculator and be very strict about the time constraints that apply in the exam.
- A useful starting point if you are 'stuck' is to try to analyse which of the arithmetical skills are needed from those that were summarised in Table 2.1 on p. 63; remember that there are only four main possibilities. Then check with the author's analysis in Section 2.7.1 and try to work out how the technique(s) identified could be applied. Only when you have exhausted every possible source of help turn to the answers and explanations (Section 2.7.2) on p. 84.

Q1 You need to make up some potassium permanganate solution, so that when 5 mL of the original solution is made up to 5 litres with water it makes a final solution of 1 in 10 000. How much powder do you need to make 500 mL of the original solution?

A ☐ 500 g B ☐ 50 g C ☐ 10 g D ☐ 5 g E ☐ 1 g

Q2 A drug is to be given at a dose of 850 mcg/m² body surface area. It is available in ampoules which contain 500 mcg of the drug per 0.5 mL. What volume of the drug must be given to an adult female of ideal body weight?

A ☐ 1.7 mL   B ☐ 2.72 mL   C ☐ 1.36 mL   D ☐ 1.5 mL   E ☐ 0.74 mL

Q3   Mrs Spencer is 70 years of age. She is extremely overweight (105 kg), and on a recent hospital visit her serum creatinine was measured as 210 micromol/litre. Her glomerular filtration rate can be calculated using the following equation:

$$\text{GFR (mL/min)} = \frac{1.04 \times (140 - \text{age in years}) \times (\text{weight in kg})}{\text{serum creatinine (micromol/litre)}}$$

Which of the following describes her renal function?

A   ☐ Normal renal function
B   ☐ Mild renal impairment
C   ☐ Moderate renal impairment
D   ☐ Severe renal impairment
E   ☐ Very severe renal impairment

Q4   What weight of a drug A, containing 10% w/w moisture, should be added when preparing a 20 litre batch of an aqueous solution formulation with a final concentration of 2% w/v of anhydrous drug A?

A ☐ 4.4 g   B ☐ 44.4 g   C ☐ 444.4 g   D ☐ 888.8 g   E ☐ 4444 g

---

Questions 5–7 concern the following quantities of sodium bicarbonate:

A   1.0 g   B   10 g   C   100 g   D   1000 g   E   10 000 g

Select, from A to E above, the correct quantity to use when preparing the following.

Q5   200 mL of Aromatic Magnesium Carbonate Mixture, BP.

Q6   4 kg of Magnesium Trisilicate Oral Powder, Compound, BP.

Q7   800 mL of a standard intravenous solution.

Q8   A female patient weighing 120 kg is prescribed six days' treatment with subcutaneous tinzaparin at the standard adult dose. What is the minimum number of vials required?

    A ☐ 2   **B** ☐ 3   **C** ☐ 4   **D** ☐ 5   **E** ☐ 7

Q9   A 1 mL vial of Stemetil injection (concentration 1.25% w/v) contains what quantity of prochlorperazine expressed in mg?

    A ☐ 15 mg   **B** ☐ 1.25 mg   **C** ☐ 12.5 mg **D** ☐ 125 mg **E** ☐ 25 mg

Q10   How many Permitabs are required to prepare 20 litres of a 0.06% w/v solution of potassium permanganate?

    A ☐ 3   **B** ☐ 30   **C** ☐ 45   **D** ☐ 300   **E** ☐ 450

Q11   A child aged four weighs 16 kg. The child is to be started on a drug at 5 mg/kg/day, divided into two doses. What dose in mg would be prescribed in the morning and evening?

    A   ☐ 20 mg morning and evening
    B   ☐ 40 mg morning and evening
    C   ☐ 60 mg morning and evening
    D   ☐ 80 mg morning and evening
    E   ☐ 100 mg morning and evening

Q12 A mixture of propylene glycol and Eumovate cream is to be prepared. The ratio of glycol to cream must not exceed 6 to 4. Suggest the formula for 250 g of the most dilute preparation that can be made.

A ☐ Eumovate cream 200 g propylene glycol 50 g
B ☐ Eumovate cream 100 g propylene glycol 150 g
C ☐ Eumovate cream 175 g propylene glycol 75 g
D ☐ Eumovate cream 150 g propylene glycol 100 g
E ☐ Eumovate cream 125 g propylene glycol 125 g

Q13 Drug A has a volume of distribution of 3 litres and an elimination half-life of four hours. What will the patient's plasma concentration of drug A be 20 hours after a 360 mg i.v. bolus of the drug is administered? (Assume linear kinetics, 1 compartment model.)

A ☐ 15 mg/mL
B ☐ 1.875 mg/mL
C ☐ 15 mcg/mL
D ☐ 3.75 mcg/mL
E ☐ 1.875 mcg/mL

Q14 What weight of netilmicin sulphate is required to manufacture a batch of 5000×1.5 mL ampoules containing 10 mg/mL netilmicin (as sulphate). Ampoules have a 10% overfill.

A ☐ 50 g B ☐ 55.5 g C ☐ 68.5 g D ☐ 75 g E ☐ 82.5 g

Q15 A doctor is insistent that he wants a dose of 7.5 mL of Ventolin SF syrup to be diluted and given as a 10 mL dose qds. He writes a prescription for a two-week supply, which the manufacturer's literature confirms is stable when diluted with water. Which one of the following do you measure out when making the diluted solution?

A ☐ 495 mL Ventolin
B ☐ 560 mL Ventolin
C ☐ 140 mL water
D ☐ 420 mL water
E ☐ 240 mL Ventolin

In questions 16, 17, and 18, answer A, B, C, D or E, where A = 1, 2 and 3 are correct; B = 1 and 2 are correct; C = 2 and 3 are correct; D = 1 only is correct; E = 3 only is correct.

Directions for MCQs Style 3 summarised				
A 1, 2, 3	B 1, 2 only	C 2, 3 only	D 1 only	E 3 only

 Q16 A pharmacist has been asked to supply three different medicines which are to be made by crushing tablets and adding a suspending agent. Which of the following instructions for their preparation is/are correct?

1 ☐ 50 mL of furosemide (frusemide) suspension 20 mg/mL: crush 2 × 500 mg tablets and make up to 50 mL

2 ☐ 300 mL of diazepam 5 mg/5 mL; crush 30 × 10 mg tablets and make up to 300 mL

3 ☐ 50 mL of spironolactone suspension 100 mg/5 mL: crush 20 × 100 mg tablets and make up to 50 mL

Q17 A local GP prescribes (at the request of a hospital consultant) the following prescription for an 11-month-old infant.

Acetazolamide 250 mg/5 mL. Suspension
Dose: 2 mL bd for 1/52
        4 mL bd for 1/52
        6 mL bd thereafter. Send 200 mL

After a discussion with 'specials manufacturing' you decide that a suitable preparation can be made with a suspending agent (that they will supply) and the crushed tablets. An expiry date of seven days is recommended. Which of the following statements is/are correct?

1　☐ The exact amount to be taken by the baby in the first week can be made using six tablets

2　☐ If only the exact amount that has been prescribed is dispensed each week, the prescription will last for at least four weeks

3　☐ After three weeks on the medication, the total daily dose of acetazolamide for the baby will be 600 mg

Q18 A pharmaceutical manufacturer wishes to market a preparation containing dihydrocodeine and paracetamol. Which of the following could legally be licensed as a Pharmacy-only (P) medicine?

1　☐ A pack of 12 tablets, each containing the equivalent of 10 mg dihydrocodeine base, 500 mg paracetamol and other excipients weighing 90 mg. The proposed dose is one tablet three times a day

2　☐ An oral solution containing the equivalent of 10 mg dihydrocodeine base in 5 mL; the proposed dose is one or two 5 mL spoonfuls twice a day

3　☐ A pack of 24 tablets, each containing the equivalent of 5 mg dihydrocodeine base, 500 mg paracetamol and other excipients weighing 90 mg. The proposed dose is one tablet four times a day

---

For each of the next two questions, 19 and 20, you will be given two statements; you then have to decide whether each statement is true or false. A further explanation of these style 4 MCQs is given on p. 133.

You have to choose an answer code as follows:

A   If both statements are true and 2 is an explanation of 1
B   If both statements are true and 2 is not an explanation of 1
C   If statement 1 is true and statement 2 is false
D   If statement 1 is false and statement 2 is true
E   If statement 1 is false and statement 2 is false

	Statement 1	Statement 2
Q19	A tablet that contains 12 mg of codeine phosphate could be classified as a P medicine if it also weighed at least 1800 mg with the other ingredients	In a tablet that contains 15 mg of codeine the percentage of codeine base is less than the ms of 1.5% if the tablet weighs 600 mg
Q20	30 mg tablets of Codeine Phosphate BP weigh 450 mg; they cannot legally be classified as a 'CD Inv P' because the ms to be a P is exceeded	A tablet containing 23 mg of codeine phosphate is classified as a P medicine if it contains less than 20 mg of codeine base as a dose

These next four questions (21–24) are a little different, as they have five possible answers (A, B, C, D and E, as before) printed before the questions. There will not necessarily be five questions, and you can use the answer codes once, more than once or not at all. These are style 2 MCQs which are explained further on p. 132.

A   Two tablets/capsules to be taken three times a day
B   Two tablets/capsules to be taken four times day
C   Three tablets/capsules to be taken three times a day
D   Three tablets/capsules to be taken four times day
E   Four tablets/capsules to be taken three times day

 Q21   The recommended dose of quinine sulphate tablets 200 mg needed to treat an adult with an unknown strain of malaria for one week is . . .

Q22 The recommended maximum dosage regimen of Ponstan capsules for an adult with period pains is . . .

Q23 The minimum dose of ibuprofen, as 200 mg tablets, to be taken daily by an adult is . . .

Q24 The maximum number of metronidazole tablets 200 mg to be taken by an adult as an amoebicide for an invasive intestinal infection is . . .

2.6   Answers to exercises

Exercise 2.1   Answers

Fraction (as the smallest number)	Part	Decimal	Percentage
Example above: 3/4	3 in 4	0.75	75
1/4	1 in 4	0.25	25
1/100	1 in 100	0.01	1
20/100 or 1/5	200 in 1000	0.2	20
2/5	2 in 5	0.4	40
1/80	1 in 80	0.0125	1.25
4/100	400 in 10 000	0.04	4
45/100 or 9/20	45 in 100	0.45	45

Exercise 2.2 Answers

	Question	Answer	Equivalent to answer in column 3
1	Dose (in mg) in 0.2 mL of an injection containing 6 mg/mL	1.2 mg	1200 mcg
2	Volume (in mL) that contains 5 mg if the injection is 15 mg/2 mL	1/3 of 2 mL	0.667 mL
3	Dose (in mcg) in 1/10 mL of an injection containing 450 mcg/mL	45 mcg	0.045 mg
4	Active ingredient (in g) in 30 g of an ointment containing 12% w/w	3.6 g	3600 mg
5	Dose (in mg) of drug at 6 mg/kg for a 25 kg child	150 mg	0.15 g
6	Mass of potassium permanganate (in g) in 250 mL of solution containing 1 part in 1000	1/4 g	250 mg
7	Volume (in mL) of an 8% w/v solution containing 40 mg	1/2 mL	500 mcL
8	Volume (in mL) of syrup to add so that a mixture containing 0.5 mg in 1 mL contains 2 mg/5 mL; 100 mL needed	20 mL	0.02 L
9	Total amount of drug (in mg) infused after two hours at 10 mg/minute	1200 mg	1.2 g
10	Total volume of solution (in mL) given at 10 drops/minute for 90 minutes if 1 drop is 0.05 mL	45 mL	0.045 L
11	% of active ingredient if a 40% solution is diluted 1 in 5	8	1/10 of 80
12	% of active ingredient if a 45% solution is diluted by taking 1 part and adding 4 parts	9	1/100 of 900
13	Volume (in mL) taken if a 15% solution is diluted to give 300 mL of 5%	100 mL	0.1 L
14	Total daily dose (in mg) of a drug given to a 7 kg baby at a level of 10 mg/kg tds	210 mg	1/7 of 1470 mg

continued overleaf

Exercise 2.2   Answers (continued)

	Question	Answer	Equivalent to answer in column 3
15	Total daily dose (in mg) of a drug given to a 20 kg child at a level of 15 mg/kg qqh	1800 mg	1.8 g
16	Total amount of drug (in g) if 250 mg given qds for one week	7 g	1/200 of 1400 g
17	Total dose of drug (in mg) at 5 mg/kg/day for 20 days to a 16 kg child	1600 mg	1/4 of 6.4 g
18	Dose (in mg) to give a 30 kg child at 20 mg/kg	600 mg	1/9 of 5.4 g
19	Number of mmol in 112 g of drug if the $M_r = 56$	2000	1/20 of 40 000
20	Volume/mL of a 0.1 Molar solution to give 5 mmol of active ingredient	50 mL	1/50 of 2500
21	The weight (in kg) of an 11 stone man. 1 kg = 2.2 lb, 14 lb = 1 stone	70 kg	70 000 g
22	The weight of cream (in g) to use for 200 g of a preparation that is base:cream in ratio of 3:2	80 g	0.08 kg
23	The weight of solid (in g) to use for 200 mL of a solution such that when diluted 40 times, a 1 in 8000 solution is produced	1 g	0.001 kg
24	The amount of drug (in mg) in 0.1 mL of a 1 in 1000 solution	0.1 mg	100 mcg

2.7 Analysis of skills and answers to MCQs

2.7.1 The analysis of skills necessary to answer the sample MCQs

Question number	Arithmetical techniques used to solve each problem					
	1 Fractions/ percentages/ decimals/ parts	2 Cancelling/ dividing	3 Scaling up and down			4 Other
			(i) Doses	(ii) Formulae	(iii) Concentrations	
1	✓			✓		✓
2			✓			✓
3		✓				✓
4	✓				✓	
5				✓		
6				✓		
7				✓		
8		✓	✓			
9					✓	
10		✓			✓	
11			✓			
12	✓					
13		✓				✓
14		✓			✓	
15	✓					
16					✓	
17				✓		✓
18	✓				✓	
19	✓					
20	✓					
21			✓			
22			✓			
23			✓			
24			✓			

2.7.2   Answers and explanations to sample MCQs

Each of the calculations will be treated in stages, i.e.

- Deciding what you know and what you need to look up.
- Converting units where necessary.
- Writing the formula so that you can scale up/down or substitute.
- 'Cancelling'.

Points to note:

- Not all the calculations will have all the stages.
- The analysis of the arithmetical skills for each sample question is given in section 2.7.1, so that it can be referred to separately to provide a clue to solving the problem.

A1   It is probably not too difficult to see that the skills of converting parts to percentages is needed. The scaling up to the formula is the last bit; the two are connected by the 'other' skill of substituting in the $C_1V_1 = C_2V_2$ formula, as are so many of these type of calculations when the parts have been converted to percentages.

(i)   **State what you know:**

$C_1 = ?$
$V_1 = 5$ mL
$C_2 = 1$ in 10 000
$V_2 = 5$ L

(ii)   **Convert to quantities so that they are in the same, manageable units:**

$V_2 = 5$ L, to be the same units as $V_1 \times 1000 = 5000$ mL

$C_2 = 1$ in 10 000, or ? in 100

Foolproof formula:

1 in 10 000
? in 100

$$? = \frac{100 \times 1}{10\,000}$$

$$= 0.01\%$$

(iii) $C_1 V_1 = C_2 V_2$

$C_1 \times 5 = 0.01 \times 5000$

(iv) $C_1 = \dfrac{0.01 \times \cancel{5000}^{1000}}{\cancel{5}_1}$

$= 10\%$ w/v solution needed

To make 500 mL, $10 \times 5 = 50$ g so the answer is B.

A2 (i) You need to look up the relationship between surface area and ideal body weight, which is on the right-hand page preceding the back cover of the BNF. It is a table that is frequently needed, so make sure you can use it accurately.

(ii) The average surface area of a female is 1.6 m^2 so the amount of drug needed is 850×1.6 mcg. There is no real alternative to the long multiplication here, but make it easier by doing 850×1.6 and not 1.6×850!
The answer is 1360 mcg.

(iii) Now the scaling up. Stick to the foolproof formula for when you know three things and need to calculate the fourth.

There is 500 mcg in 0.5 mL
So there is 1360 mcg in ? mL

so $? = \dfrac{1360 \times 0.5}{500}$

Divide carefully by 5

   = 1.36 mL

Answer is C.

A3   **(i)**   The level of renal impairment is measured by calculating the GFR – see Appendix 3 in the BNF for the definitions. A different skill, that of substituting in a formula, is therefore needed, and then some cancelling.

      (ii)   Thankfully, all the numbers you have been given are in the same units as the formula, so no conversions are needed.

      (iii)   GFR (mL/min) $= \dfrac{1.04 \times (140 - \text{age in years}) \times (\text{weight in kg})}{\text{serum creatinine (micromol/litre)}}$

$$= \frac{1.04 \times (140 - 70) \times (105)}{210}$$

At first glance, the sum looks impossible, but don't despair. Solve the bits in brackets first and then, if you have been working on your 7 times table, you should spot that the numbers above will cancel (there are lots of other ways too) to give:

$$= \frac{1.04 \times \overset{1}{\cancel{70}} \times \overset{35}{\cancel{105}}}{\underset{1}{\cancel{210}}}$$

GFR $= 1.04 \times 35$ mL/min

Again, do the easy long multiplication (i.e. 35×1.04) to give a value of 36.4 mL/min, which corresponds to mild renal failure, so the answer is B. Or you could have made the whole question a lot easier and just used the creatinine clearance value of 210 micromol/litre which was given!

A4   **(i)**   Not much!

(ii)   Convert 20 L to mL; multiply by 1000 = 20 000 mL.

(iii)   To have a final concentration of 2% of the anhydrous drug A, extra must be added to allow for the moisture it contains.

1 g in 100 mL is 1% w/v

2 g in 100 mL is 2% w/v
  ? g in 20 000 is 2% w/v

$$\frac{?}{2} = \frac{20\ 000}{100}$$

$$? = \frac{20\ 000 \times 2}{100}$$

$$= 200 \times 2 = 400\ g$$

but for Drug A, that will contain 10% water and only 90% of drug.

400 is 90%

  ? is 100%

$$\frac{?}{400} = \frac{100}{90}$$

$$? = \frac{100 \times 400}{90}$$

= 444.4 g or answer C.

A5   **(i)**   From the BNF, Aromatic Magnesium Carbonate Mixture, BP contains 5% sodium bicarbonate.

(ii)   200 mL contains 10 g; as 5% means 5 g in 100 mL, the amount to be used is double = B.

A6 **(i)** From the BNF, Magnesium Trisilicate Oral Powder, Compound, BP contains 250 mg per gram of sodium bicarbonate.

(ii) The only possible difficulty here is converting 4 kg to grams, but even that is not really needed, as 250 mg is $\frac{1}{4}$ of 1 g, then the answer must be $\frac{1}{4}$ of 4 kg or 1 kg, which is equivalent to 1000 g or answer D.

A7 **(i)** From the BNF, the standard intravenous solution contains 1.26%.

(ii) In 100 mL, there is 1.26 g, so there is 8 times as much, which equals 10 g. Answer = B.

A8 **(i)** From the BNF, the standard adult dose differs for prophylaxis and treatment of deep vein thrombosis; the appropriate dose is 175 units/kg/day. The vials contain 40 000 units.

(ii) The dose is 175 units/kg, so for a weight of 120 kg, the dose needed for six days = $175 \times 120 \times 6$ units.

(iii) Which is a nasty long multiplication; however all is not lost! You need to calculate how many vials are needed; each contains 40 000 units, which you need to divide by:

$$= \frac{175 \times \cancel{120}^{3} \times 6}{\cancel{40\,000}_{1000}}$$

now you can cancel and simplify the sum: divide by 10 and by 4, but not by 2 as well; it's easier to divide by 1000 than 500.

$$= \frac{175 \times 3 \times 6}{1000}$$

$$= \frac{3150}{1000}$$

= 3.150 vials.

As you cannot dispense a part vial the answer must be 4. Answer = C.

A9   (i)   The only piece of information you are given that you can work from is that Stemetil injections contain 1.25% w/v of prochlorperazine.

(ii)   Care! The basic statement is in grams, the answer in mg. Probably best to convert at the end, but could be done in the first line.

(iii)   There are 1.25 g (or 1250 mg) of prochlorperazine in 100 mL. So there is ? g (or mg) in 1 mL.

(iv) $$\frac{?}{1.25} = \frac{1}{100}$$

$$? = \frac{1 \times 1.25 \text{ g}}{100} \quad \text{or} \quad ? = \frac{1 \times 1250 \text{ mg}}{100}$$

= 0.0125 g or 12.5 mg

so the answer is C.

A10   (i)   What are Permitabs? From the BNF, you find that they each contain 400 mg of potassium permanganate – they feature here as another variation on the theme of dilution calculations!

(ii)   Convert litres to mL, i.e. 20 × 1000 = 20 000 mL needed. Watch the Permitabs too.

(iii)   There is 0.06 g in 100 mL, so there is

? g in 20 000 mL

$$\frac{?}{0.06} = \frac{20\ 000}{100}$$

$$? = \frac{20\ 000 \times 0.06\ g}{100}$$

but as each Permitab contains 400 mg, you can divide by that quantity to convert the sum to a number of tablets. But you need to convert them to grams as well, as the final quantity is in grams, so multiply by 1000 too all in the one calculation. (In case you don't follow why, you are effectively dividing by the fraction 400/1000. The rule remembered by some from primary school days is 'to divide by a fraction you turn it upside down and multiply!).

(iv) So the number of Permitabs = $\dfrac{20\ 000 \times 0.06 \times 1000}{400 \times 100}$

cancel by 10 by 4 and by 2

= 30 or answer B.

A11 **(i)** All the information is given; a typical example of the necessity to read the question carefully.

(ii) The child needs to take 5 mg/kg/day. The dose per day therefore is 5 × 16 = 80 mg. So the answer is B – easy if you read the question carefully.

A12 **(i)** Another one to read very carefully! The ratio of glycol to cream that is the most dilute is 6:4.

(ii) The whole sum is very much easier if you use the ratio 3:2 not 6:4.

(iii)   As 250 g is needed, and the total number of parts 2 + 3 = 5, it is not too difficult to see that each part is 50 g, so the ratio of glycol to cream is 150 g: 100 g. As the answers are written the other way round, it is all too easy to choose answer D, but the cream to glycol ratio is 3:2; you want it the other way round, i.e. answer B.

A13   (i)   Don't panic! We haven't had one like this, but the information you need is all there: i.e. linear kinetics and the length of the half-life. There is a formula to work it out, but without a calculator, its use is not recommended. No – it's back to basics and halving the quantity for each half-life time until 24 hours has elapsed.

(ii)   This is where the complication comes in; the answers are in mcg/mL or mg/mL. The units given for concentration are mg in 3 litres.

(iii)   At time 0, the concentration is 360 mg in 3 litres. After four hours, the concentration halves to 360/2 = 180 mg in 3 litres. After eight hours it halves again and so on, until five half lives have elapsed. The amount of drug therefore goes 360/2 = 180/2 = 90/2 = 45/2 = 22.5/2 = 11.25 mg.
To convert to the quantity per litre, you need to divide by 3, so there are 3.75 mg/L. To convert to the quantity per mL you have to divide by 1000, and to convert mg to mcg multiply by 1000.

(iv)   The two cancel each other out, so the answer is 3.75 mcg/mL or answer D.

A14   (i)   Although it looks a bit complicated, this is a simple scaling up of a formula, once you have calculated the total final volume.

(ii) The answers are in grams, the information in mg, so there will have to be a conversion at some point.

(iii) First of all, calculate the total volume needed, which is 5000×1.5 mL + 10% for the overfill

$= 5000 \times 1.5 = 7500$ mL + 10% = $7500 + 750 = 8250$ mL

There is 10 mg in 1 mL,

so there is $?$ mg in 8250 mL

$$\frac{?}{10} = \frac{8250 \text{ mg}}{1}$$

$$= \frac{8250 \times 10 \text{ mg}}{1 \times 1000}$$

$= 82.5$ g or answer E.

A15 (i) This is another example that has not been met before, but has all the information you need; there is no need to know the concentration of the Ventolin syrup, for example.

(ii) The total volume of solution to be dispensed is $10 \times 4 = 40$ mL per day, $\times 14 = 560$ mL for a fortnight. As 7.5 mL represents $\frac{3}{4}$ or 75% of the dose volume, it must be the same proportion of the total volume: i.e. $\frac{3}{4} \times 560 = 420$ mL Ventolin and 560–420 mL = 140 mL water (or, of course, 25% of the total).

Answer is C.

A16 *Statement 1*

50 mL of furosemide (frusemide) suspension 20 mg/mL: crush 2 $\times$ 500 mg tablets and make up to 50 mL

The amount needed is 20 mg/mL, so for 50 mL, 50 × 20 = 1000 mg, so 2 × 500 mg = 1000 mg is correct.

Statement 2

300 mL of diazepam 5 mg/5 mL; crush 30 × 10 mg tablets and make up to 300 mL

The amount needed is 5 mg/5 mL.

so ? mg in 300 mL

$$\frac{?}{5} = \frac{300}{5}$$

$$? = \frac{300 \times 5}{5}$$

$$= 300 \text{ mg}$$

which is the same as 30 × 10 mg tablets, so the statement is correct.

Statement 3

50 mL of spironolactone suspension 100 mg/5 mL: crush 20 × 100 mg tablets and make up to 50 mL

Need 100 mg in 5 mL,

? mg in 50 mL

i.e. multiply 100 × 10 = 1000 mg, so statement is incorrect, as 20 × 100 mg tablets = 2000 mg.

Answer is B.

A17 This is an example from practice, so don't think it can't happen to you! It is a real example of analysing and evaluating, too. If you look up the only tablets that contain acetazolamide (Diamox) first, you find the clue to the whole problem.

Statement 1

The exact amount to be taken by the baby in the first week can be made using six tablets

Statement is false.

The tablets contain 250 mg each; consequently for a 250 mg/5 mL suspension, six tablets makes 30 mL. It doesn't take long to work out that 2 mL bd for 1/52 is 28 mL. In practice you would make a volume that uses a whole number of tablets and label it with the expiry date and an instruction to discard any remainder.

Statement 2

If only the exact amount that has been prescribed is dispensed each week, the prescription will last for at least four weeks

Statement is false.

You have already calculated that you need exactly 28 mL for the first week, so for double the dose, double the quantity will be 56 mL. In the third week the volume is $12 \times 7 = 84$ mL. Total so far is 168 mL; another 84 mL will make the total volume more than 200 mL, so the last installment in the fourth week will have to be for less than the full amount – the prescription lasts for less than four weeks.

Statement 3

After three weeks on the medication, the total daily dose of acetazolamide for the baby will be 600 mg

This is true.

Volume is now 6 mL bd = 12 mL od. 250 mg in 5 mL, so 250/5 × 12 = 600 mg.

Answer is E.

***

For questions 18–20, it is essential to use the MEP. This question tests your understanding of the CDs that can be CD POM, CD Inv POM or CD Inv P. The legal classification of these drugs depends on the limiting factor/s of maximum strength (ms), the maximum dose (md) and/or maximum daily dose (mdd). For a detailed explanation, refer to Level 1 question 9, in *Practical Exercises in Pharmacy Law and Ethics* (Appelbe, Wingfield and Taylor).

A18   *Statement 1*

For single dose preparations, ms must be < 1.5% and md < 10 mg; no mdd or limit on pack size.

10 mg as a percentage of the whole weight of the tablet is

$$\frac{10 \times 100\%}{10 + 500 + 90} = \frac{1000}{600} = 1.67\%$$

Cannot legally be a P.

Statement 2

For undivided preparations, ms must be < 1.5% and md < 10 mg.

$$10 \text{ mg in 5 mL as a percentage} = \frac{10 \times 100}{5} = 200 \text{ mg/100 mL}$$

i.e. 0.2% – OK as less than 1.5%, but md is 10 mg; as a dose of one 5 mL spoonful contains 10 mg base and the dose is one or two 5 mL spoonfuls, which contains 20 mg of dihydrocodeine, it cannot legally be P at that dose.

Statement 3

Again a single dose preparation; % will be approximately half of the amount from statement 1, as it is 5 mg not 10, so 0.875%; dose is one tablet, so well under the md of 10 mg, so could legally be sold as a P medicine.

Answer = 3 only or code E.

A19 *Statement 1*

For a 'single dose preparation' of codeine (i.e. a tablet) to be a P medicine, the ms (as base) is 1.5% w/w, and the md has to be 20 mg. A dose of 12 mg is alright, provided that it does not exceed 1.5% of the mass of the tablet, which is 1800 mg.

The percentage of codeine is therefore

$$\frac{12 \times 100\%}{1800}$$

cancel by 100 and by 6 = 2/3 = 0.667%.

So the statement is true (if you are wondering why such a preparation is not available, think of the possible implications, not least of which is how big the tablet would have to be!).

Statement 2

15 mg as a percentage of 600 mg is

$$\frac{15 \times 100\%}{600}$$

cancel by 100 and by 3 = 5/2 = 2.5%.

The statement is false. The answer overall is therefore C.

A20   *Statement 1*

30 mg as a percentage of 450 mg is

$$\frac{30 \times 100\%}{450}$$

cancel by 10, 5 and 3 to give $\frac{20}{3}$, which is clearly more than the ms of 1.5%,

so the statement is true.

Statement 2

You might think that this is true; you don't need to (indeed can't) calculate the actual amount of codeine base but the condition concerning the ms also applies and so the statement is false.

Answer = C.

A21   The recommended daily dose of quinine sulphate tablets 200 mg needed to treat an adult with an unknown strain of malaria for one week is 600 mg of certain quinine salts, of which the sulphate is one, every eight hours, so the answer is C.

A22   The recommended maximum dosage regimen of Ponstan capsules for an adult with period pains is 500 mg three times daily, so the answer is A, as each capsule contains 250 mg.

A23   The minimum dose of ibuprofen, as 200 mg tablets, to be taken daily by an adult is 1.2 g in three or four divided doses, and the tablets contain 200 mg each, it must be six tablets a day or two tablets three times a day so the answer is A.

A24   The maximum number of metronidazole tablets 200 mg to be taken by an adult as an amoebicide for an invasive intestinal infection. The BNF gives a dose of 800 mg every eight hours, which is equivalent to four 200 mg tablets three times a day, so the answer is E.

2.8   Summary

Hopefully you are now in a position to understand why calculators are not allowed in the registration exam, and you have also gained some insight into the reasons for the decision. For many pre-registration trainees, the exercises and sample calculation questions will be a valuable part of their exam preparation and revision. However, there are many other aspects worthy of consideration, and the next chapter examines them in more detail.

❸

Be prepared!

3.1   Introduction

If your first response to the idea of preparing for the registration exam is to ask 'Where do I start?' the quick answer is – it's impossible for someone else to say! Each candidate will have a different perception of what they need to do, and how they achieve their aim will of course vary too. Consequently, the following guidelines can only be suggestions; ultimately, it is up to each individual to decide on their own course of action. However, if you have had difficulties with exams and the revision for them in the past, perhaps now is the time to do some *preparation* first. If the italics in the previous sentence need an explanation, it's to emphasise that there are important differences between 'exam preparation' and 'revision'. Basically, preparation covers all the things you need to do to be in a position to start revising. A good example would be doing some of the exercises in Chapter 2, where you might have identified the need to learn a new skill, and then practise using it. Revision involves going over what you have learnt – perhaps by doing some more questions. The two activities will be treated separately so that you can identify which is your priority, and to give you some constructive ideas.

Even though every preregistration trainee will have successfully undertaken many exams before, the registration exam is different – both in the format of the exam and especially in the significance/implications of failure. It represents the culmination of many years of effort and is quite rightly perceived to be the final hurdle in a long struggle. It is therefore hardly surprising that even graduates who have previously taken examinations in their stride start to panic as the great day approaches. It doesn't make any difference when those who have seen them progress from undergraduates to mature (almost) professionals offer reassurance; the prospect of failure is too awful to contemplate but still ever-present. There is always a 'scaremonger' who 'knows' that the questions will be different/impossible/demand hitherto unheard of feats of memory – and worse.

The only answer that a bystander can give at this point to the mass hysteria generated amongst groups of preregistration trainees is to ensure that they are as well prepared as possible, both throughout the year and for the exam itself. Most trainees will be perfectly capable of organising themselves in terms of completing the entry forms, preparing and following a revision timetable and even collecting the appropriate resources. However, for this exam there are other features for which even the most confident candidates may well need some support and encouragement. For less well-organised mortals, some of the more basic hints, preparation ideas and revision tips that follow might make the difference between failure and success. Whilst there is no substitute for ongoing preparation throughout the year, all preregistration trainees should find something extra here to help them in the analysis of the syllabus and what it means in terms of the questions that are set. Needless to say, the rest is up to the individuals concerned.

3.2   Comforting facts to remember/refer to in moments of crisis

The title of this section says it all.

- On average, 90% of those who attempt the exam pass first time.
- Only 37 candidates who graduated in the UK out of the many thousands who have taken it have failed to pass after three attempts and have not been able to register as a pharmacist.
- When you leave the exam room, the only questions you remember are those you found difficult to answer; you forget the vast majority that you answered correctly.
- If the answer to a question is contentious or ambiguous, or

the statistical analysis reveals a large number of alternative answers, then the question may be removed from the total mark, which will improve everyone's score.

- Your undergraduate exams were designed to test whether or not you were able to demonstrate sufficient knowledge and skills to graduate in the relevant discipline, not whether or not you have developed the additional qualities necessary to practice as a pharmacist.

- The aims of the assessment procedures used by universities will often apply to many different courses and are bound to be quite different from those set by the Pharmaceutical Society, with the responsibility to regulate standards within the profession.

- The pass mark of 70% over the total of 170 questions means that 30% or 51 questions can be wrong and you'll still pass (so long as you also manage to get at least 14 out of the 20 calculations questions correct).

- A lot of the knowledge needed for the exam is developed during the preregistration year, which means that all the time you have been working, you have also been preparing. As this is such a vitally important concept not only to the whole ethos of the year but for you as a worried preregistration trainee, it is discussed in more detail below.

- And finally – according to at least one preregistration tutor:

If you have been working systematically through your RPSGB training material and programme, no revision should be necessary. The only preparation needed is to acquire a good working knowledge of the reference sources to be used in the exam.

3.3 Using the syllabus to your advantage

However, for those who may doubt the wisdom of that last statement, and want to prepare themselves and then revise as thoroughly as possible, read on. Having recognised that no one else can tell you what to do, or when to do it, there is, however, an obvious starting point – and builds upon the point made earlier about the interdependence of both aspects of the assessment programme in achieving overall 'competence' to practice.

The overall aim of the registration exam is to test that you, the newly qualified pharmacist, will be able to put into practice the skills, knowledge and understanding that you have acquired during the last year in order to practise effectively and independently. That means that exam needs to test you in two main areas:

- Can you demonstrate you have the knowledge needed?
- Can you apply that knowledge to practice?

3.3.1 Knowledge

Taking the first point, the exam must assess whether or not you have gained the knowledge and understanding of the core topics necessary for effective practice. The topics in the syllabus that form the 'core of knowledge' have been decided upon as the result of many discussions between experienced pharmacists from all branches of the profession. However, the other knowledge requirements indicated in the syllabus and what is tested where and how also needs to be incorporated into exam preparation. The use of performance indicators rather than the term 'competence' indicates that it's not just the list of topics in the registration examination syllabus that is needed. The requirements for registration also include a 'working knowledge' that you must have in order to be able to perform appropriately – the principles of professional decision making is a good example.

3.3.2 Application

However, for an examination that permits you to practice independently as a professional, the possession of a body of specialist knowledge and a working knowledge of other skills is not enough.

You need – no, *have* – to be able to demonstrate that your knowledge can be used to interpret new situations and other problems met in everyday practice. Educational experts have been involved to ensure that the style of the exam meets that demand, hence the reference to the analysis and evaluation of practice-based problems and the use of the term 'learning outcomes' in connection with the core topics. The implications of what those terms mean for the questions with which you are presented and how to prepare for them are discussed briefly here as what it means to be able to apply your knowledge.

Think back to your undergraduate exams, or A-levels, for a moment. Did you ever come out of an exam and complain that you had never heard of the chemical that the question was about? Or have to work out what a new drug, with a known chemical group, might do in the body? Those questions are the sort that ask you to apply your knowledge in a new situation, and are considered by many to be a far better test of how you would perform in an unfamiliar setting than the conventional 'learn the lecture notes and regurgitate all you can remember' essay question. Although that is an over simplification of a complex topic, the skills being tested in each situation are quite different. Whilst each type of exam question has its place, those that assess the 'application of knowledge' and need a 'problem-solving' approach are far more appropriate to the practice of pharmacy. The ideal is also reflected in the overall character of questions, which is covered in more detail in section 4.2.

There is one very comforting thought to consider now, in terms of your exam preparation. Remember that the key element of the whole programme is experience; as you work with others you will be supported in your learning by doing and by evaluating what you have done. But of course you, as ever, have a vital role to play in all aspects of your learning and exam preparation. If you think about it, you will begin to realise that the more you take the opportunity to learn at all times, the more opportunities you will create to apply your knowledge – and prepare for the exam. Let's take a final example to make the point crystal clear. You are doing the labels for a prescription and notice from the PMR (patient medication record) that a new drug has been added. Let's say it's a patient who takes warfarin and she is prescribed a low dose of aspirin. Your knowledge – and no doubt the software and the BNF – will tell you that there is an interaction which is potentially very serious. It's no good going out to the patient and telling her 'there's an interaction between your new medicine and your warfarin' and proceed to tell her all about protein binding and volumes of distribution. That's the specialist knowledge that you have, that tells you the interaction can be very serious – and also might have been included in the detailed answer the lecturer wanted in the graduation exam. Neither can you hide behind others for too long, although of course your tutor will want – and need – to be involved. In order to demonstrate that you can act professionally and apply your knowledge, you have got to consider very carefully all the reasons why the prescriber might have wanted the two together – or not, as the case may be. Then you have got to decide what to do before you talk to the patient, who is waiting. The way you apply your knowledge in such a difficult situation demands a very different set of skills; acquiring them is what the preregistration year is all about. The moral of the tale being – don't just let labelling be the task you are doing – use it as a learning opportunity and you will be able to provide evidence of many aspects of performance standard A1 (for those on the new course) *and* a knowledge of professional decision making *and* prepare for the exam!

Perhaps the remark by the tutor was accurate after all – anyway, it's hopefully apparent by now that the more you put in towards demonstrating and applying your knowledge and acquiring skills in the practice situation, not only will it enable you to meet the necessary standard of appropriate skills, but also to prepare for the exam.

3.4   Translating the syllabus into questions

However clear and helpful a study of the aims and objectives appears to be, there are still many preregistration trainees who need further reassurance that they have interpreted the intentions of the examiners correctly. Their understandable concerns do not usually arise from the format of the exam or the implications of the other relevant information. What they really want to know is how the list of topics that comprises the syllabus is translated into actual questions that will (realistically, it can only be 'could') be asked. The common queries are presented below; examples to illustrate important points are taken from the sample questions already published, and from some new questions.

How up to date do I have to be?

The syllabus for the examination was first published in 1992, and was the result of a long consultation process with many of those involved in preregistration training. Since then, several revisions have taken place to reflect changes to practice, and to encompass suggestions made by tutors, members of the Council of the RPSGB and also from the examiners. Details of the original syllabus and subsequent changes have been reported in the Journal and are not a matter of concern in the present context. Any agreed updates are introduced at the beginning of the training year and are included in the copy of the syllabus sent to all preregistration trainees; further vital information is sent individually in the form of two bulletins from the Education Division. The obvious intention of the examiners is to make the syllabus reflect recent changes in practice and current educational aims for the assessment of a work-based postgraduate experience.

There are also some constraints imposed by the examining process which can be an advantage to candidates. The questions are drafted some time in advance of both the summer and autumn exams; consequently, the reference sources on which the questions are based have to be those current at that time. Any publications printed after the exam questions are drafted, even if they are updated versions of textbooks that are needed for the open-book paper, could contain information that is not expected/given as a possible answer. A question may therefore be set for which the answers given are out of date, according to an article that you have read recently. In such an instance – and they have occurred – it is likely that when the answers are statistically analysed, there will be clear evidence of the understandable confusion, and the question will be eliminated from the final calculation.

A word of warning: In previous exams, it was quite possible to rely on the information sources available at the beginning of the academic year and the fact that they could not be updated. With the advent of the use of the Internet to access parts of the syllabus such as 1.11 (b) – aspects of NHS legislation with relevance to pharmacy – it would be wrong to rely on resources that might well be out of date when compared with the 'online' version. With the NHS changing so rapidly, it has always been an area which is difficult to examine, especially at the application of knowledge level. Again, there will have to a 'cut off' point at which further change is not examined; no doubt that will be clearly communicated to preregistration trainees.

Where do I find the information I need?

An obvious exam preparation activity is to study the topics listed in the syllabus and check that you have appropriate information about each of them. Some of the units will inevitably cause problems if you only refer to undergraduate notes. The most likely reason/s for omissions are:

- The topic was not on the undergraduate syllabus.
- It was on the undergraduate syllabus but not covered in sufficient depth.
- It was taught, but not related to what is needed for practice;

remember that the aims and some of the content of the under-graduate and preregistration syllabi are completely different.

An example will make the point more clearly. Consider the case of the hospital preregistration trainee who realises that s/he does not know much about the products needed for 2.1.(c), 'Non-Prescription Remedies,' and who does not have the opportunity to work in a community pharmacy as part of his or her training. In many schools of pharmacy the use of over-the-counter (OTC) drugs and products is only mentioned very briefly – after all, the degree course has to accommodate knowledge about a huge range of potent drugs. The logic with regard to OTC drugs is often that anyone who needs to know about them (i.e. those going into community pharmacy) will learn about the current remedies and preparations in their preregistration year. The registration exam syllabus quite rightly makes the sale of OTC remedies a significant part of the clinical practice requirements. Anyone who does not sell them every day needs to find out about the products and, of course, the theories of 'differentiating minor illness from more serious disease' (2.1.(d)) as part of their exam preparation.

A solution to the problem described above is to use the recommended reference sources. You are expected to complete the CPPE package 'Responding to Symptoms' and have access to any of the following textbooks in the pharmacy: *Symptoms in the Pharmacy: a guide to the management of common illness* (Blenkinsopp and Paxton), *Non-prescription Medicines* (Nathan) or *Minor Illness or Major Disease?* (Edwards and Stillman). They will all include the listed topics in sufficient detail to answer the exam questions. Another approach is to use a reference source that includes most of the necessary topics; the most appropriate recent publication is the second edition of *Pharmaceutical Practice* (Winfield and Richards). Probably an even better idea is to use all the sources mentioned, to ensure that you have covered the topic thoroughly – which emphasises the difference between, and the importance of, exam preparation and revision. If you do not have a suitable reference source to work from, you will not be able to revise. The only way you can do that is to spend some time well in advance of the exam studying the syllabus and selecting the topics for which you need additional material, and then make sure it is acquired. It might mean that you have to order some textbooks, as they may not be available at your local library. Access to the Internet will undoubtedly help here too – so long as you are sensible about the amount of time spent 'surfing'.

You can perhaps see that the process of preparation for revising for this exam is not quite as straightforward as for undergraduate exams – where, generally, little preparation was needed, as you could depend on revising from your lecture notes, handouts, and the university library nearby, to get you through.

What depth of knowledge is needed?

A great many preregistration trainees worry about the depth of knowledge needed, especially in unfamiliar areas. Well-meaning pharmacists with whom they work might well add, perhaps unintentionally, to the sense of unease that is experienced. For example, a recently qualified pharmacist who has also completed a Clinical Diploma will have at their fingertips a wealth of knowledge and skills that you, as a newly qualified member of the profession, are not expected to possess. Equally, a practitioner of 20 years' standing could also mislead you; if their clinical knowledge is out of date, they might well feel intimidated by the amount you can remember – and tell you that it will not be needed!

The main information you are given about the depth of knowledge needed is again in the reference books already referred to and your knowledge of what is needed in all areas of practice. There is also some useful guidance given in the examination guidance notes. For example, the level of knowledge that is needed of the Data Protection Act is only as it applies to pharmacists in the context of their practice – when using a PMR system, for example. A much more thorough working knowledge is quite rightly expected of the laws that you will constantly need to apply as central to the practice of pharmacy – the Medicines Act is an obvious example.

Further comfort with regard to exam preparation can be derived from briefly repeating several relevant points:

- The registration exam is for non-specialists – it is the same for everyone.
- It does not depend on the knowledge and experience gained by either someone who has done a Diploma or a practising pharmacist even one year after registration.
- The type of examination and the knowledge tested are different from undergraduate exams – the aims reflect the need to develop professionalism.
- Topics that go out of date quickly are only set to test knowledge and perhaps comprehension; the 'higher-level' (and consequently more difficult) skills are not tested.

In summary, it should now be obvious that successful exam preparation, and hence revision, takes:

- time;
- planning;
- money.

But think of the necessary expenditure as an investment in your future!

3.5 Some tried and tested hints for exam preparation

Successful candidates have made the following suggestions to help you with your exam preparation and revision. Use those that apply to your individual circumstances.

3.5.1 Months/weeks before the exam

- Make sure you have and understand all the available information about the structure of the exam.
- Book a week's holiday for the beginning of June.
- Identify known exam weaknesses and work on them.
- Read and understand all sections of the syllabus and order any textbooks needed.
- Obtain reference sources for the open-book exam a.s.a.p. – possibly buy the BNF.
- Flag/personalise/annotate the open-book reference sources and use them when you are at work (refer to the Workbook/manual and the May bulletin to ensure that exam regulations are not contravened).
- Don't spend ages on less important bits and the bits you know you know.
- Do CPPE packs and learn the NHS legislation a.s.a.p.
- Do company 'projects' etc. a.s.a.p.
- Arrange a mock exam using the sample questions.
- Arrange to work with other preregistration trainees sometimes.
- Do all the activities that are not in your specialism and check off as many performance standards as soon as possible, e.g. the principles of responding to symptoms, and knowledge of the Drug Tariff for hospital candidates.
- Use a pocket notebook for unfamiliar/new drugs and brand names, especially for OTC preparations.
- Cut out updates from the Journal – for example drugs/preparations that change from POM to P.
- Transfer/duplicate information in the bulletin to a separate exam folder – it means less panic and saves time looking later.
- Calculations – make a note of each 'everyday' example and do them as you are working (that of course is the intention of the exam) without a calculator.
- Send in your entry exactly as instructed.
- Practice the 'turn to' test, as described on p. 16 as often as possible.

3.5.2 Days before

- Check entry documents that you need to take.
- Organise travel to the venue.
- Organise overnight accommodation if necessary.
- Check the exact route and parking arrangements.
- Choose whom to meet beforehand and don't get side-tracked into talking to colleagues/'friends' whom you know will 'wind you up' before exams.
- Check reference books, pencils, rubbers, etc.

3.5.3 The day before

- Make sandwiches/something to eat for the next day and buy drinks; there's a lot of hanging around beforehand, and not much time to get out to buy lunch between papers.
- Do something to try and take your mind off the next day – suggested activities ranged from the unprintable to 'arrange a hard game of squash/football/whatever to ensure you sleep' to 'go to the mosque/church/whatever is appropriate and pray'.

3.6 Some tried and tested exam revision hints

So – your preparation is in place, you have all the information and textbooks needed, and the reference books for the open-book paper are flagged, highlighted and annotated. You have organised your entry, travel arrangements and whom to meet. What do you actually do next? Revise. Yes, but how, for such a different type of exam?

A few initial words of caution/explanation in case you feel that your tutor is not as helpful as you had hoped in your exam preparation. For a start, there is no better example of the importance of taking responsibility for your own progress than in your preparation and revision for the exam. Whilst tutors are very involved in your day-to-day assessment, they will in many cases not have had the 'experience' of the registration exam and perhaps may feel ill-prepared to offer advice. In other words, it's definitely up to you – again.

If the above point is obvious, the next one – that no one else can do the revision for you – is probably even more superfluous. Candidates for the registration exam will have developed their own revision techniques, which have already been successful. Consequently, there is no attempt in this section even to begin to describe the different methods that can be used for revising, other than to make the general point that revision should involve an activity – that means doing something to relieve the monotony of going over previously prepared notes. If the activity means making new notes, referring to textbooks and new material – it is probably preparation rather than revision, which is simply going over information and material previously understood and memorised. Another vital revision activity is doing past papers/questions, but again that needs to be done in such a way to extract the maximum advantage from the exercise. By now, you might well ask, if current practitioners are not going to be able to help with revision what other possible contenders are there to offer advice? The answer is to refer to those who really can be constructive – those who know because they have succeeded. Preregistration trainees from the last few years were asked to list points concerning the exam and its revision that they thought would help. Amongst those who commented were two who failed the first time around – a salutary experience, but one from which you can benefit. The points are listed in no particular order, and are written as the candidates described them, with a few explanations. Several of the points raised are considered in more depth in Chapter 4.

3.6.1 General points about revision

- Make a timetable and stick to it.
- Create a grid listing your essential tasks/topics, etc. and when you plan to tackle them.

- Be realistic about revising after work.
- Throw away most university notes.
- Do your own thing – summarising notes, chanting, sample questions, etc. – you know what helps by now.
- Work with another preregistration trainee if that helps – but choose wisely.
- Be prepared.
- Start in plenty of time.
- Unlike when you're at university, you have to go to work all day, every day – use holiday time wisely.
- Throughout the year, make a note if something unknown arises and set time aside to do it.
- Don't question pick – they're all compulsory.
- Arrange a 'we're not going to panic' meeting.
- Listen to/use the ideas of others, e.g. their essential preparation activities.

3.6.2 Brief points about exam technique

Many topics are also covered in more depth in Chapter 4.

- Eliminate obvious wrong and poor 'distracters' – guess from less.
- Remember that some combinations of answers are not allowed.
- Check carefully or highlight anything negative and anything in bold writing.
- Remember every word in the 'stem' of the question counts, e.g. *serious* ADR.
- Know enzyme inducers and inhibitors to work out interactions.
- Likewise, know the hierarchy of which drugs are plasma protein bound, so what will be displaced by what and the consequences of high levels of each, e.g. digoxin, lithium.
- Do a 'mock' exam, but remember that a paper lasting one hour is not that good a preparation; each 'real' one is much longer, and you get very tired.

- The 'mock' can give a false sense of security, especially if you have seen many of the questions before.
- The exam is very clinical – you have plenty of time in the 'mock', but not in the real one.
- Don't 'flag' the entire BNF, but do flag cardiovascular drugs, the beginning pages and sections – too many flags are counter-productive.
- Do Style 4 'assertion: reason' questions (at the end of each paper) first, before you get completely tired and confused.
- The English of the questions is often harder to understand than the content.
- Guess quickly once the obvious wrong answers have been eliminated.

3.6.3 Comments from two candidates who failed the first time around

- Don't rely on dispensers/technicians/counter assistants to answer queries – look them up yourself.
- Make your tutor test you.
- Make other pharmacists test you.
- Make a plan.
- Get going sooner.
- Know important and uncommon adverse drug reactions (ADRs).
- Use the information from the Society concerning your performance to plan the retake. Do not ignore such data as your percentile score – it can be used to your advantage.
- Get all the coaching/hints/help that you can.
- Learn from your mistakes.
- Use those who have taken it/others judiciously – the exam has changed.

3.7   Exam procedure

The following comments have been supplied by a recent group of (successful) candidates.

3.7.1   Beforehand

- Make sure that your mail reaches you promptly – a designated drawer in your workplace is vital, plus a reminder to all staff to use it!
- Check your exam centre's code number against the actual location; one student was given one centre, but the code indicated that he was expected at another. If a similar or other mistake happens, chase it at once.
- Use exactly the same name on all degree certificates, submissions to the RPSGB, etc. Any differences may not be picked up until the registration procedure, and then it means a worrying and expensive trip to the solicitor to do a 'statutory declaration' rather than concentrating on your revision.
- Check the bulletins carefully – all the information you need about forms and dates is there! If you move to another location, you will need to chase them – they're vital.

3.7.2   On the day itself

- If you possibly can, stay near the exam centre. Some companies organise and pay for a block-booking for candidates, which is greatly appreciated. Apart from removing the worries about travelling to the centre and traffic delays, it gives everyone the chance to discuss last-minute concerns and to support each other.
- Be aware that centres tend to differ in their interpretation of the regulations for exam registration. At one you are told to report an hour before the start, but you don't get to sign in and have your photo checked, etc. straight away – there's a lot of waiting. When you are registered, you have to go to

your desk inside the hall and wait again – very nerve-wracking. At another centre, photos are checked when candidates are sitting at their desks doing the exam.

- Be prepared for delays; at most centres there are 150+ candidates, so inevitably a few difficulties arise organising so many people. If there is more than one room being used, you will need to consult a special notice-board to find out which one you are to be in.
- Don't forget to take the evidence of your candidate number – you will need it for the morning and afternoon registration.
- Don't take anything that beeps – all mobile phones and watches, etc. are put onto a table from which you can only hope to collect your belongings later.
- If you do not receive your notification about the exam, contact the organisers at once or it may be too late. It should come three weeks beforehand – to the day.
- The gap between exams is about right; canteens are available for those who feel able to face lunch.
- It's a very long day, as you don't finish until after 5 p.m.

3.7.3 Content of the exam

General

- The RPSGB sample papers issued in May are very similar in standard to the 'real' exam, although the content is different. You can get a false sense of timing – the real ones takes much longer – but doing them as a 'mock' is good practice.
- The clocks in the exam room may be different – don't think you have two minutes longer than you actually have.
- The time goes really quickly, and, at the end, you don't know how you've done. In a university exam, you usually know whether or not you have managed the 40% pass mark, but when it's 70%, it's impossible. You only remember the questions you couldn't do, so don't discuss them afterwards.

A few final words from immediately after the exam

- The closed-book paper consisted of the simple, obvious and downright impossible; don't be despondent – two wrong answers won't fail you. You can get 30 wrong on this paper and still pass.
- There's lots that you need to know about – read widely throughout the year. NB after the 2000 examination, the examiners were concerned that questions on diabetes, nutrition and contraception were answered badly. Part of your preparation should perhaps include some extra work on these topics.
- Some topics that are generally less well known concern stability, sterility and excipients.
- Plan to do the open-book paper as closed-book.
- If you don't know – make an educated guess.
- Do those you can, improve your confidence and go back to the harder ones.
- The obscure questions are not hard – just obscure.
- The exams are both very 'clinical' – you use the BNF a lot for the open-book paper.
- Some of the questions which are set to test your knowledge of the *Drug Tariff* are better answered using the BNF; for example, which bandages are allowed – this information is indicated towards the back of the BNF (in Appendix 8) but it is very difficult to find in the *Drug Tariff*.
- Some of the sample questions tended to be ones that you either knew or didn't, whereas lots in the 'real' one can be worked out/manipulated. This is especially true of law and ethics questions and reflects the information on the syllabus – that the questions set will be practice-based with the main emphasis on the skills of evaluation and application.
- If you are almost certain about the answer, respond without looking it up. Put a mark to indicate that you'll check later if there is time. You don't have time to look through the Medicines, Ethics and Practice guide – you have to know where to look, or forget it!

- There were some questions on nutrition, which was an unknown topic to many and reflected the availability of the new reference book (Mason). Similarly there were many on response to symptoms, again based on the new edition of a recognised reference source (Blenkinsopp). Everyone said that such questions were straightforward.

Hopefully you will be able to use some of the advice given during your own exam preparation and revision programme; there's nothing as good as evidence from a primary source – except when it's from more than one!

4

The exam questions – analysed, audited – 'sorted!'

4.1 Introduction

In Chapter 3 the meaning of exam preparation was explored, and some hints and activities that others have found helpful were considered. It was recognised that even the best candidates might not have thought of some of the ideas mentioned, as the registration exam is so different from all those previously undertaken.

With the preparation activities (hopefully) going well and the revision about to start, any consideration of the techniques to be used raises additional difficulties. Generally, methods vary so much that any attempts to offer advice must either be non-specific or tailored to the needs of each candidate – which is beyond the scope of this 'survival guide'. However, there is one very important aspect of revision – analysing past questions – that is a particularly appropriate activity, and can be recommended to all preregistration trainees. But isn't that a contradiction of what has just been stated? As graduates who have been conditioned to think, it's likely that many preregistration trainees will ask 'why' in response to such a suggestion. Why is an analysis recommended when other revision techniques are left up to the individual? What is special about such an analysis, and, more to the point, how can it help everyone? These are all very good questions, and deserve detailed answers. In order to emphasise yet again where the responsibility for learning lies, the information is considered very much in terms of what you, the individual preregistration trainee, can do to help yourself.

Before thinking about whether or not you need to be involved, have another look at the title of this chapter. Even if you are not quite sure about the exact difference between the terms 'analysis' and 'audit', hopefully the (colloquial) use of the word 'sorted' attracts your attention sufficiently to read on. Think about it – assuming that you have 'sorted' the ongoing activities that will enable you to meet the other criteria for registration, it is now only your revision methods and exam technique that stand between you and your certificate. Consequently, the general idea of this chapter is for you to improve your exam technique to a point where enough of the questions can be answered correctly, in the time available, for you to pass the exam. In other words, the questions are also going to be 'sorted' – in both senses of the word, as you will see.

However, instead of just establishing what type of question is asked most frequently, on which topics and at what depth (called an analysis), that information is going to be used further in order to improve your exam performance (known as an audit). As the principles of audit and its role in improving practice are now a topic that are included on the exam syllabus, a practical application of the process is even more appropriate as a revision activity. An alternative title for this chapter could well have been 'Improving your exam technique by analysing questions' – but how many of you would have thought 'I don't need to know any more about that – I've already passed all sorts of exams' – and missed it out? Yet again, the different nature of the exam should lead you to think that perhaps there are some unusual features that necessitate a more careful study of the possible techniques to employ in order to pass.

If you were astute enough to notice the earlier anomaly, you have no doubt also spotted another major difficulty. In order to perform a detailed analysis of previous questions, as suggested above, there should be some complete past papers available. Before you get really hopeful – there aren't. Although sample questions and other information are published, the Society does not release whole papers to anyone, and an analysis of the sample questions would be meaningless. Instead, the general information about the exam and the character of the questions will be analysed and then audited. The process and its significance have been summed up in Fig. 4.1.

Looking at each of the numbered stages in turn, there's not much you can do about the need to pass the exam (stage 1) as one of the criteria for registration, and the standards that have been set

Figure 4.1   A suggested audit of performance with respect to the registration exam. Adapted from p. 463 of *Pharmaceutical Practice* (Winfield and Richards).

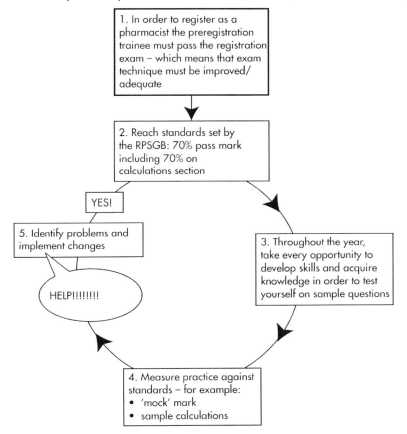

to do so (stage 2). If you have been working effectively throughout the year, you will have undertaken lots of learning activities in the course of your daily duties, and can complete stages 3 and 4 by taking responsibility for your own learning. For example, if you have completed the self-audit of your skills, or the diagnostic calculations, you will be making a very good start. If you then take steps to improve your performance or develop new skills by completing some activities that you or your tutor have agreed might help, then you really are doing as much as possible to identify problems and implement changes (stage 5). For some, this stage is the one that causes problems, as they either cannot be objective enough in identifying their problems, or, more commonly, do not know where to start to implement changes. Unless you are able to measure yourself again against the same standards, you don't know if you have done enough to ensure that you pass, which is where further difficulties are liable to occur. What if your 'mock' mark is lower than that of your friends and/or does not reach the magic 70%? What if you do not get 70% on the section on calculations? What can you do to improve your score? What if you know that you had problems on the open-book paper, because you haven't met one before? Where do you start? Again, the onus is very much on you doing something to help yourself – which is where the audit that follows can act as a constructive part of your revision as it will help you to know where to start. Once you know what your problems are, then hopefully there will be a section in this book to help. If you are now at the stage of trying to be objective about what to do next now that you have not done as well as you had hoped to, the following sections are designed to help you know where to start.

4.2 An audit of the idiosyncrasies of the registration examination

For each of the following inherent characteristics and distinctive 'features' of the registration exam, the possible implications for all candidates are examined. You will then be in a position to audit your own performance against each one, and decide which of the points apply to your circumstances. Consequently, you'll be in a better position to implement appropriate changes in order to adapt or improve your exam technique and performance. As some of the 'features' that follow involve a consideration of aspects of the syllabus and examination using unfamiliar terminology, these are summarised very briefly first.

4.2.1   A summary of the structure and terminology

- The final examination will consist of two papers which contain a total of 170 multiple choice questions (MCQs).
- For the open-book paper (Paper 2) you are expected to have and use (judiciously), the three reference sources which are arguably the most commonly used in the practice of pharmacy.
- For the closed-book paper (Paper 1) there are no reference sources available.
- Each style of MCQ will be in a block of similar questions with instructions as to how to answer them. The chosen answer code must be clearly marked on an answer sheet with a soft pencil; it is then 'computer read' and your score calculated.
- To achieve the aims of the exam, a combination of four different styles of MCQs are used which:
  - Test for four different skills/capabilities (knowledge, comprehension, analysing and evaluating).
  - Are perceived to be at one of three levels of difficulty by the examiners.
- A minimum of 20 calculation questions are included on the open-book paper, although it is possible that reference sources will not necessarily be needed for all of them. It is also possible that other questions on both papers will involve further calculations.
- Other than an emphasis on questions focused on allowing graduates to demonstrate the skills of analysing and evaluating practice-related problem-solving situations, there is no further indication as to how many questions will be set from each of the above categories. It is probable that the relative numbers of each type of MCQ will vary between the open- and closed-book papers.

4.2.2 Unusual features and their possible implications for candidates

Feature 1:

The examination consists of two papers, which take place in various centres on the same day in late June. The 'resit' exam, which is also the first exam for many, is held in late September

Implications

● You will need to check the exam regulations, the syllabus and other information sent to you directly and in the form of bulletins so that you know all the relevant facts about the administration of the exam.

● The large number of candidates entered at each site means that there are associated difficulties with registration, including a lot of waiting about, which can make you even more nervous.

Feature 2:

The *second* paper (Part 2) is an 'open-book' exam

Implications

● The open-book paper is now held *after* the closed-book one. The timing has changed to try and prevent those candidates who didn't finish the open-book paper being too upset to do their best on the closed-book paper, which was previously held in the afternoon.

● It is a particularly appropriate style of examination, as it mimics exactly what happens in practice – namely that it is not so important to know and/or remember the vast amount of information that a pharmacist needs to have at their fingertips, but rather that it is a much more appropriate skill to be able to look up effectively and efficiently, as explained in detail in Chapter 1.

● If you haven't done an open-book exam before, you perhaps won't realise one of the fundamental differences in the approach – namely that the exam is not easier because the books are there. On the contrary, the questions often refer to little-known drugs/groups of drugs and to exact details for which you have to search diligently.

● The skills that are tested mean that the questions are very different – they are set in such a way that you often have to refer to the books, which takes time. Although there are fewer questions (80) on the open-book paper than on the closed (90), there is only 150/80 or 1.875 minutes on average for each one.

● In Chapter 1 the recommendation that no more than 1 hour out of the 2.5 is spent on the calculations was considered. If you are not confident, or take a long time to do the arithmetic, there is a severe danger that you will spend too long on this section, still get a few wrong, and not complete enough of the other questions.

● Combine the difficulties with calculations and the more complex questions, where there is more than one statement to consider, and you can see that you will not have sufficient time to flip idly through the reference sources in the vain hope of stumbling on the right bit of information. (When students invariably complain that they didn't have enough time to finish an open-book exam, they are referred to the anecdote concerning the monkeys, the typewriters and the writings of Shakespeare. The theory being that if there is enough time, one of the monkeys will eventually reproduce the complete works of the Bard! Whilst not really suggesting that there is any comparison between graduates and monkeys, there is some truth in the analogy – which is why the time is strictly limited.)

● The books to be used are three well-known reference sources that you must not only take to the exam, but with which you must be totally familiar, or you will not finish. Consequently, your exam preparation must include practice at finding the types of information which are most frequently asked for – that means 'flagging' the sections that you consider to be important, for example.

- Most candidates, including those who have done open-book exams before, will agree that by far the best practice is to do sample questions from the Society and any others relevant to the aims of the exam that you can find, under exam conditions. In the new programme, sample questions are likely to be very limited, as those previously circulated contain questions set on topics that are no longer on the syllabus. Another worry is the inclusion of new topics for which there are very few, if any, sample questions.

- Another pitfall is to refer to the book because it is there, even when you know you know the answer – it acts as a security blanket but wastes time.

- A final very useful piece of advice from a successful candidate – if you are 95% certain of the answer, don't look it up to be sure – mark your response on the answer sheet and indicate somehow that it's one to return to if there's time. You have to make time to consider all the questions first.

Feature 3:

Both papers consist solely of multiple choice questions

Implications

- There are some advantages, including the fact that the correct answer is given, and as there is no negative marking, guesswork may get you the mark.

- Also, there is no need to worry about writing, spelling, punctuation etc. – you simply mark, in pencil, the chosen code on a 'computer read' answer sheet. There is no (possibly subjective) marking by a tired/bored examiner – the computer is always correct and fair to everyone. It is also used to analyse statistical information about the responses.

- Of course, there are obvious disadvantages too. You may find that none of the answers is quite right, or the question appears ambiguous, which you cannot explain in your answer to the examiner. There is no chance to do well on one question to make up for others – each scores one mark, however hard you work to get the answer. As you are not physically writing the answers, the examiners expect the time to be spent thinking/working instead. Consequently, the questions often demand that a lot of complex information has to be read and understood before even thinking about the answer – which is very tiring, especially towards the end of the second paper. However, perhaps you can see the relevance to practice emerging – the thinking is called 'cognitive processes', which might make you feel a little better.

- There is no chance to 'question pick' – every question is compulsory, and a great deal of the syllabus can be covered in a single examination.

- Although your final percentage score comes from the overall mark on both papers, the statistical analysis can be used to extract information about which questions were answered well, and those that you answered incorrectly. Of course, the new exam from 2002 will also include the analysis of the calculations section.

Feature 4:

There are four different styles of multiple choice questions

Implications

- It is not necessary to understand the rationale for the different styles of questions or how the combinations are used to meet the objectives of the exam; it is important to be prepared to respond appropriately to each.

- The instructions for answering the particular style of question are given in full at the beginning of the section of similar questions and repeated on each double page thereafter; it makes sense to refer to them rather than guess at the code for a particular style/combination. It would be very unfortunate to work out the correct answer and then fail to get the mark because you remembered the code wrongly.

- The relative proportions of each style of question is not fixed, but generally there are fewer of the more demanding ones (Styles 3 and 4 below). With the advent of an even greater emphasis on the skills of analysis and evaluation, which are perhaps easier to assess by the use of MCQ styles 3 & 4, it is possible that the proportion of these might increase.

- The RPSGB does not publish exact information about either the number of questions to be set at each level of difficulty (as assessed by the examiners and item writers) or how many of each style of MCQ are included. However, the syllabus does state that 'overall, the main emphasis will be on application and analysis/evaluation' – which is, of course, the most appropriate to assess whether or not a candidate can provide an effective pharmaceutical service.

- Further vital information and some general points about the four individual styles of question and how to answer them are considered in more detail below. The points made under the heading 'Pitfalls/playing the system' are each given a reference code so that further relevant features of the questions can be considered later. In order to understand the language of MCQs, note that the question is known as an 'item', the possible answers the 'lettered options' or 'codes', and the introductory statement or question the 'stem'. For Styles 1 and 2 there have to be possible answers which are incorrect, otherwise known as 'distracters'.

Feature 5:

The nature of the exam demands that questions are set to enable the desired exam objectives and assessment goals to be achieved

Implications

The syllabus describes the topics for which you need to demonstrate your knowledge and understanding in order to satisfy the examiners that you can practise effectively and independently. However, as has been mentioned before, the way that you will need to demonstrate your knowledge is likely to be somewhat different from, say, an undergraduate exam.

It is the additional, higher level (harder) skill of being able to apply that knowledge to a new situation that therefore has to be tested. Although that may sound a bit hard, remember that that is what you have been doing throughout your preregistration year – the exam is only testing what happens in practice. The fact that many of the questions will ask you to analyse and evaluate practice-based scenarios rather than just being asked to recall the relevant knowledge is not only entirely appropriate, but also familiar.

4.2.3 The multiple choice question styles investigated

Style 1: Simple completion (SC)

Directions: Each of the questions or incomplete statements in this section is followed by five suggested answers. Select the best answer in each case.

Which means: There are five codes given, A, B, C, D and E. Choose the one that best answers the question or completes the statement, even if you don't fully agree with any of them.

Pitfalls/playing the system

SC1.   The description and directions for Style 1 make these questions – of which there are lots on each paper – sound easy. Not necessarily so! When well written, each of the distracters is so nearly right that you might be taken in, especially on a topic about which you are not very sure.

SC2.   However, for every right answer there are four that have to be wrong – which can be used to your advantage. The distracters are often the hardest to write; they need to be plausible, and not too obscure. Look for an obvious misfit that is there to make up the numbers – which can quickly be discarded as a possibility. If you are going to have to guess – which is always a justifiable possibility when the answers are given and there is no negative marking – at least make it an educated one. The whole ethos of chance in a professional exam seems inappropriate, but if you have demonstrated at least some knowledge and skills in eliminating those answers that you know are incorrect, then the use of educated guess work can (grudgingly) not only be justified, but helpful. Also remember the point made in Chapter 3, that the pass mark of 70% over the total of 170 questions means that 30% or 51 questions (assuming that you have the minimum 70% on the calculations) can be answered wrongly overall and you will still pass.

SC3.   Another obvious point about exam technique that is well worth repeating: if you must guess, don't spend ages doing so. On the open-book paper especially, time is very tight, and you must give yourself a chance to have a go at all the questions – there may be lots later on that you will find easier.

SC4.   Look carefully at every word in the stem; the question writer and the reviewer will have done so, and you can be sure that everything is there for a reason, even if it is not immediately apparent from the first question. Sometimes several items are grouped together (the numbers are always clearly indicated), and then a detailed piece of information is given, or a scenario is described, on which the relevant items are based. Note that the answers are not sequentially dependent on each other (that would mean if you got the first one wrong, you would also get the others in the group wrong too, which is patently unfair). It is just that all the information for the group of items is given together. For each item, go back to the stem and read it all again – the vital information you need is there, even if it appears at first that more is included than necessary.

SC5. While on the subject of the importance of single words, always look out for give-aways like 'must', 'should' and 'could' in the options – they are often mutually exclusive, in that if you 'have' to do something, it cannot be a recommendation too. The imperatives are much less appropriate in questions on the Code of Ethics, for example.

SC6. Other points about exam technique that you have heard many times before are still just as relevant, plus a few variations on the theme:

- Read the question – the use of negatives and exceptions to the rule completely alters the question that is being asked – and of course the answer you must give.

- If you must mark each code on the question paper with the intention of transferring them to the answer sheet before the end, make sure that you leave enough time to complete the task, and to check the accuracy of your transfers. Generally, everyone recommends that you answer questions on the final sheet as you decide on them.

- Mark the items that you are not sure about so you can come back to them later if you have time, but get at least an educated guess onto the answer sheet in the meantime.

- Do the section containing the question style that you find most difficult first, when you are relatively fresh. In the open-book paper this will probably be the calculations, or the section of Style 4 questions in both papers.

● Don't forget to prepare the reference sources, pencils, rubbers, etc. that you are taking to the exam, in plenty of time.

Style 2: Classification (CL)

Directions: Each group of questions below consists of five lettered options followed by a list of numbered questions. For each numbered question select the one lettered option which is most closely related to it. Each lettered option may be used once, more than once, or not at all.

Which means: There are five codes given, A, B, C, D and E, one of which is the correct answer to each of the range of questions (i.e. numbers 9–11, for example) stated. However, that doesn't mean that the same answer cannot be given twice – it can! Indeed, all the questions could have the same answer, which means that not all the codes will be used.

Pitfalls/playing the system

CL1. Treat each question on its merits – don't be influenced by the previous answer.

CL2. The only difference to Style 1 questions is that the five possible answers are given once before the questions, and apply to the range indicated. Consequently, the same principles apply – for example, all the possible answers should be applicable to each question; if not that could well be a clue as to the answer, as in SC2.

Style 3: Multiple completion (MC)

Directions: For each of the questions below, ONE or MORE of the responses is (are) correct. Decide which of the responses is (are) correct. Then choose:

A   if 1,2 and 3 are correct

B   if 1 and 2 only are correct

C   if 2 and 3 only are correct

D   if 1 only is correct

E   if 3 only is correct

Directions for multiple choice questions Style 3 are summarised below:

Directions for MCQs Style 3 summarised				
A 1, 2, 3	B 1, 2 only	C 2, 3 only	D 1 only	E 3 only

Which means: There's a lot more work to do to get the one mark allocated, as you have to look at each of the responses to decide if it is a possibility. You cannot stop when you have found one that's correct – they all could be.

Pitfalls/playing the system

MC1. Learn the forbidden combinations of lettered options – you cannot choose just 2, or 1 and 3. If you think either of those choices is the answer, you need to look very carefully at all the words in the stem again – perhaps you have missed a vital clue.

MC2. Don't run the risk of getting the right answer but the wrong code – check the directions each time.

Style 4: Assertion: reason (AR)

Directions: The following questions consist of a statement in the left-hand column followed by a second statement in the right-hand column.

Decide whether the first statement is true or false. Decide whether the second statement is true or false. Then choose:

A   if both statements are true and the second statement is a correct explanation of the first statement

B   if both statements are true but the second statement is NOT a correct explanation of the first statement

C   if the first statement is true and but the second statement is false

D   if the first statement is false and the second statement is true

E   if both statements are false

Which is then summarised on each page of questions below:

Directions for MCQs Style 4 summarised			
	First statement	Second statement	
A	True	True	2nd statement is a correct explanation of the 1st
B	True	True	2nd statement is NOT a correct explanation of the 1st
C	True	False	
D	False	True	
E	False	False	

Which means: There's even more work to do to get the one mark allocated.

Pitfalls/playing the system

AR1.   As they are difficult to write and very testing to answer, only a few examples are included on each paper. They are, however, likely to continue to be used, as they particularly test problem-solving and evaluation skills.

AR2.   The section that contains them is always at the end of the paper. Some candidates recommended doing them first, whilst still relatively fresh.

AR3.   Remember that the use of true and false statements limits the use of the 'best' answer used in all the other styles of question; there is no degree of suitability to be judged, just a clear-cut yes or no – which means that many clinical situations cannot be examined, and that, if you know your law, a false statement is easy to spot. There are also many instances of the words 'advised' and 'recommended' in the Code of Ethics and Practice Advice – which means a question that says you 'must' do something is false.

AR4. Each of the statements that constitute a question must not only stand alone as a grammatically correct entity but also as one that could possibly be connected to the other. The temptation is to write two unconnected statements, which would reduce the number of possible codes that are considered. It is also very difficult to write plausible false statements, so overall there tend to be fewer D and E answers.

AR5. The difficulty most frequently encountered is deciding between codes A and B, where both the statements are true but it is not obvious whether or not the second one explains the first. A good way to help you to decide is to put the word 'because' between the two statements.

4.2.4   A brief investigation into the use of different question styles

The four skills to be tested

As has already been mentioned, in order to test your knowledge and understanding, and the ability to apply it, four different skills or abilities are assessed using the four styles of MCQs described above. The four skills to be assessed are presented below, with the official RPSGB interpretations of what each means.

1. Knowledge – the ability to recall and communicate information as well as specific facts, this may include recall of terminology, techniques, theories and so on.

2. Comprehension – the ability to interpret familiar information. This is a routine level of understanding. The solution of problems and calculations in a manner with which the candidates are familiar would fall into this category.

3.   Application – the ability of candidates to use and communicate their knowledge and understanding in situations which, to some extent, are unfamiliar or to deal with familiar situations by unfamiliar methods.
4.   Analysis/evaluation – the ability to analyse a complex communication or situation into its various parts and to see the relationship between them, compose a communication, bringing together several areas of knowledge and understanding and forming a statement complete in itself.

Pitfalls/playing the system

It is quite possible that at least most of the exams you did at university (and for A-level) contained a more 'traditional' type of question than those used in the registration exam. In the former, the questions do not go beyond asking you to recall information, and then to present it in the form of an essay. If that's the case, you will be at a serious disadvantage when meeting problem-solving MCQs for the first time unless you incorporate sufficient preparation into your revision plans. As in so many instances, the principles are best explained in the form of examples. Each question is used here to illustrate a single point, and have many other valid reasons for use in the university or alternative context.

Examples of question types other than MCQs to test relevant skills

All the sample questions that follow are to demonstrate the points about the different skills and how they are tested; they are on the general topic of 'sale and supply of medicines' which is section A1.11(a) of the syllabus. The chosen topic addresses the learning outcome 'You must be able to demonstrate an understanding of: the legal requirements for the sale and supply of medicines and controlled drugs from pharmacies'.

1. A possible essay question

What are the requirements of the Medicines Act when supplying Prescription Only Medicines to the public in an emergency?

In order to answer the question, you would have to list the requirements, which can be learnt; there is no need to understand what happens in practice, or to apply what you have learnt.

2. Possible short answer question

List five requirements of the Medicines Act when supplying a POM to a member of the public in an emergency.

This is a shorter version of the essay question, testing the same knowledge but no other skills.

3. An alternative possible short answer question – spot the difference

A pharmacist interviewed a regular customer who had lost his salbutamol inhaler; the customer was wheezing badly and frightened he would not be able to get another one. The surgery was shut, so the pharmacist decided to supply a replacement.

Consider the above scenario and then answer the questions that follow:

(a) Which Act controls the supply of Prescription Only Medicines to the general public?
(b) Describe very briefly the type of supply that was made by the pharmacist.
(c) In your own words, give two further questions that the pharmacist should ask before the supply could legally be made.

The difference, when you have the two questions to compare, is hopefully quite clear. By introducing a scenario, the skills of comprehension, application and even analysis and evaluation can be tested too – which makes the item practice-based and problem-solving. This is a much more appropriate manner in which to assess preregistration trainees, but less suitable for undergraduates with no experience of practice. The next section looks at how the approach can be maintained using MCQs.

The use of the four styles of MCQs to test the four skills

The same section of the syllabus is used for the examples that follow; in many cases, the knowledge needed is very basic, so try to treat the questions as 'closed-book'. If you are really not sure, then do them as open-book items, before referring to the answers in Section 4.2.8 (see Table 4.2). Also note that at least some of the questions have deliberate errors, to highlight the points mentioned earlier; they too are explained in the answers.

Learning Points Questions 1–3 are Style 2 items; choose one of the answers A–E as the most appropriate description of the supply that is described.

A   Emergency supply at the request of a patient
B   Emergency supply at the request of a doctor
C   Supply exempt from the controls on retail sales
D   Wholesale supply to a professional
E   Retail sale to a member of the public

Q1   A pharmacist supplies a research group at the local university with some insulin for use in laboratory experiments. The necessary legal constraints are met.

Q2   A local doctor is in the pharmacy; he wants a supply of Co-proxamol tablets to carry in his bag. He has run out and will undoubtedly need some to supply to patients when he is 'on call' tonight.

Q3   A local doctor telephones you on a Saturday afternoon from a patient's house; he has just discovered that the regular monthly supply of insulin that was dispensed last week has not been put in the fridge, so he has told the patient not to use it. Can you arrange for a replacement supply as soon as possible?

Learning Points Questions 4 and 5 are Style 3 multiple completion items.

Which of the following statements is/are correct?

1   Wholesale supply
2   Supply exempt from the controls on retail sales
3   Retail sale

Q4   A local optician is on the phone; she wants to know if it is possible for you to supply her with some tetracaine (amethocaine) eye drops. She has dropped the last bottle and needs them for an eye test booked today.

Q5   A dentist is in the pharmacy; he and his wife are on holiday in the area and she has left her blood pressure tablets (atenolol) at home. You agree that the supply can be made to the dentist. What type of supply, from those mentioned, can be legally be made in the scenario described?

Learning Points Questions 6 and 7 are Style 4 multiple choice questions on emergency supplies.

	Statement 1	Statement 2
Q6	A doctor can legally request any medication that is classified as a POM to be supplied to one of his patients, in an emergency, even if they have not had the medication before	If a patient requests a supply of a POM medication in an emergency, they must, as a legal requirement, have been prescribed it in the last six months, unless it is for a seasonal product for hayfever, for example
Q7	If a doctor requests that you supply a patient with a medication that they have not had before and promises that he will supply a prescription tomorrow, that would be not be an illegal request under the Medicines Act	A requirement of the Medicines Act for an emergency supply at the request of a doctor is the need to 'furnish a prescription within three days'

4.2.5 Coping with different levels of difficulty

In order to provide a suitable range of questions to test candidates appropriately, the decision as to whether the item is hard, average or easy has to be made by the question writer and considered again by the reviewer and examiners. Although both pharmacists and the educational experts involved will be very experienced in their field, they are not thinking in terms of how hard the item is for practising pharmacists with ten years' experience, but considering the level at which the average preregistration trainee works. Another important point is that the exam is the same for all, in whichever area of practice you have spent most of your time.

4.2.6 Previously issued sample questions: a different analysis

In the section that follows, an analysis of sample MCQs from a variety of sources, including the previously issued RPSGB open- and closed-book papers, is performed. Although most of the following questions were set according to previous syllabuses, the examples chosen are used to summarise a few more exam hints and make relevant points. Note that many of the questions test know-ledge, not how it is applied, and that they are not very often practice-based or problem-solving. The somewhat unusual classifi-cation and 'sorting' of questions each has a particular purpose/learning objective/educational point to make. Reference to previous points are made using the abbreviated question style numbers allocated. In addition, the author's perception of the level of difficulty and the skills to be assessed are presented in Section 4.2.8 on p. 150, together with the correct answer code and a brief explanation.

The intention of this section is to encourage candidates to look at MCQs from a different perspective, which will enable them to meet the demands and unusual features of the registration exam in an informed manner. If they can demonstrate such qualities as the ability to 'problem-solve' and apply appropriate knowledge in unusual situations successfully, then they will pass the exam – which is undoubtedly the short-term aim of every preregistration trainee. From the information provided about the exam, it is obvious that the Society also considers these qualities to be vital, in order to be able to cope with the demands of practice and provide an effective pharmaceutical service.

Easy question: don't waste time looking up

Previously issued sample question 1

Q1   Which of the following drugs may cause gynaecomastia?

A   ☐ Bromocriptine
B   ☐ Cimetidine
C   ☐ Levodopa
D   ☐ Erythromycin
E   ☐ Diazepam

Previously issued sample question 2

Q2 A breast-feeding mother comes to your pharmacy and requests an analgesic. Which one of the following analgesics should be avoided?

A ☐ Paracetamol
B ☐ Ibuprofen
C ☐ Syndol
D ☐ Aspirin
E ☐ Propain

Easy question: poor distracter – eliminate early

Previously issued sample question 3

Q3 Which of the following 'black-listed' items can be prescribed generically?

A ☐ Benylin Expectorant
B ☐ Contac capsules
C ☐ Cytacon liquid
D ☐ Dulco-lax tablets
E ☐ Nulacin tablets

(If you are not aware of the term 'black list,' it is the term used when restrictions to NHS prescribing were first introduced, nowadays known as Part XVIIIA of the *Drug Tariff*.)

Previously issued sample question 4

Q4 Which one of the following statements is correct about the recommendations that can be made for non-prescription sale?

A ☐ Ibuprofen can be recommended as an alternative analgesic in a patient sensitive to aspirin
B ☐ Daktarin (miconazole) gel 15 g can be recommended for the treatment of a baby with oral thrush

C ☐ Codeine linctus can be recommended for a chesty, productive cough

D ☐ Aspirin can be recommended for a headache in a 10-year-old child

E ☐ Hydrocortisone 1% cream can be recommended for napkin rash

Content unknown: don't panic – think logically and rely on reference source

Previously issued sample question 5

Q5 A doctor has prescribed oral rehydration salts and wishes to provide 12 mmol of sodium (Na^+) and 18 mmol of glucose. Which of the following would most closely meet his requirements?

A ☐ Electrolade 5 sachets

B ☐ Rehydrat oral powder – 1 sachet

C ☐ Dioralyte effervescent tablets – 2 tablets

D ☐ Dioralyte oral powder – 5 sachets

E ☐ Dioralyte Relief – 2 sachets

Previously issued sample question 6

Q6 Which of the following is allowed on an NHS prescription?

A ☐ Communion wafers

B ☐ Cobalin 1000 mcg/mL Injection

C ☐ Cod Liver Oil BP

D ☐ Cephos powders

E ☐ Copholco cough syrup

Absolutely no idea: guess – no point in returning

Previously issued sample question 7

Q7   What is the Pharmacy Healthcare scheme?

A   ☐ A textbook on response to symptoms

B   ☐ Department of Health policy for pharmacists

C   ☐ A series of leaflets advertising pharmacy services

D   ☐ A series of leaflets on health topics available through pharmacies

E   ☐ An organisation looking after the health of pharmacists

Previously issued sample question 8

Q8   Normal body temperature, in °C, when taken by mouth is:

A   ☐ 35.2

B   ☐ 36.8

C   ☐ 37.7

D   ☐ 38.2

E   ☐ 38.6

Whole question depends on seeing the significant word in bold

Previously issued sample question 9

Q9   Which of the following is **not** in the list of minimum requirements for computerised patient medication records?

A   ☐ Patient age

B   ☐ Patient name

C   ☐ Medical practice name

D   ☐ Quantity of drug supplied

E   ☐ Patient telephone number

Previously issued sample question 10

Q10   A customer comes into the pharmacy and asks for something to treat his cough. On further questioning, which of the following symptoms **alone** would result in the recommendation to see a doctor?

1   ☐ The cough is associated with shortness of breath
2   ☐ The patient has had the cough for three weeks
3   ☐ The cough is in a child eight years old

Prejudicial/unknown words

Previously issued sample question 11

Q11   A drug which obeys a first-order one compartment model assumes:

1   ☐ An increase in the rate of elimination with increasing steady state serum levels
2   ☐ Instantaneous distribution following intravenous dosing
3   ☐ A biexponential decay profile for logarithmic concentration versus time

Previously issued sample question 12

Q12   Under the provisions of the Health and Safety at Work Act 1974, pharmacy managers must ensure:

1   ☐ Adequate maintenance of machinery
2   ☐ Safe transportation of dispatched articles and substances
3   ☐ That relevant training and information procedures are provided

4.2.7   Demonstrating the pitfalls of multiple choice questions

The last part of the analysis of idiosyncrasies that you can use to audit and improve your exam technique contains some new questions written to demonstrate some of the pitfalls of question writing that you can use to your advantage (see Table 4.1), including the special difficulties associated with assertion: reason (Style 4).

NB Where appropriate, read the statements with and without the bits in brackets. Are your answers the same?

Table 4.1 Demonstrating the pitfalls of multiple choice questions

Demonstrating pitfalls	Statement 1	Statement 2
Q1	If a new medicine was produced containing 100 mg/5 mL of codeine, it would legally be classified as a CD Inv POM/ Schedule 5 CD	The six CDs that can be placed in Schedule 5 include codeine
Q2	A young man, who is in the area to compete in an important football tournament, can safely be sold tablets containing chlorphenamine (chlorpheniramine) for his cold (he does not take any other medication)	Anyone who has hypertension is recommended to avoid (systemic) sympathomimetics as they cause vasoconstriction
Q3	A pharmacist who is called to a patient's house during the working day to deal with a faulty oxygen cylinder can still be considered to be in personal control of the pharmacy, even though P medicines cannot be sold in his absence	If a pharmacist leaves the dispensary to attend to a casualty outside the shop he cannot supervise the sales of P medicines
Q4	A pharmacist working in health promotion at a secondary level is likely to be working with groups of people already diagnosed with an illness or suffering early symptoms of the disease	Health education at a tertiary level could involve the individual counselling on the use of a nebuliser given by a pharmacist to a patient, in order to try and prevent his asthma becoming even worse

4.2.8 Answers and explanations to questions

This section provides the answers and explanations to the questions that have been posed throughout the audit (Section 4.2). If you have been reading each bit in the hope of being able to identify where to start in order to improve your exam technique, this is the bit that enables you to check your understanding of the point being made, and act accordingly.

See Table 4.2 (p. 148) for answers and explanations to Learning Points multiple choice questions (Section 4.2.4).

See Table 4.3 (p. 150) for answers and explanations to previously issued sample questions: a different analysis (Section 4.2.6).

See Table 4.4 (p. 152) for answers and explanations to Demonstrating pitfalls multiple choice questions (Section 4.2.7).

4.3   Concluding remarks

If you have worked carefully through the analysis, and taken your time to understand the points made about the intentions for the exam, you should now be in a position to audit your exam technique, identify problems and have some ideas as to how to eliminate them. The final activity in your exam preparation is to practise doing sample questions. In Chapter 5, a further selection of new questions is included, together with suggestions on how to answer them.

Table 4.2 Answers and explanations to Learning Points multiple choice questions

Skill being tested K = knowledge C = comprehension A = application E = analysis/evaluation

Level of difficulty H = hard A = average E = easy

Question number	Answer code	Skill being tested	Level of difficulty	Reason
Q1	C	A	A	The university does not supply the insulin, or administer it to humans in the course of their experiments, which are the definitions of wholesale supplies. (If that were the case, a registered doctor would have to apply to carry out a clinical trial.) It is a retail sale, but exempt from the legal restrictions for selling POMs. PLUS SC2, SC4 – laboratory use – and SC5. If it's wholesale it can't be retail. Poor question.
Q2	D	A	A	It fulfils the criteria for a wholesale supply mentioned in question 1 – check in the MEP. Same points apply.
Q3	B	A	E	Although the supply was made to the patient, it is the doctor requesting the whole amount to be replaced, presumably by means of a new prescription. SC2: as insulin is now a POM, you can quickly eliminate E, and D is also not valid. Unfamiliar situation, hence application.
Q4	B	E	H	A lot to think about here, especially as it's not a common request; definitely an open-book example – but there is hope. Remember the statement about 'mutually incompatible' distracters? Well here's a deliberate one. If a supply is retail, it cannot be wholesale as well – which this obviously is. Search carefully and you will find that she is allowed to purchase these, in an emergency, to administer, not supply, and that it is also exempt from the restrictions on the control of some POMs. All that definitely means it is testing skills at the highest level – analysis and evaluation.
Q5	B	E	H	Slightly less complex and less obscure than question 4, but still evaluation rather than comprehension. It is legal because a dentist can, theoretically, prescribe any POM, which is then exempt from the controls of retail sale and a wholesale supply if you supply him. Whether or not the supply is ethical is very much open to question. In practice it would be much better to do an emergency supply to the patient. The name of the drug is included because if the blood pressure medication were not a POM, it would be a retail sale. Also 1 and 3 not allowed – a poor question.

Table 4.2 (continued)

Question number	Answer code	Skill being tested	Level of difficulty	Reason
Q6	E	C	A	Statement 1 is false – all CDs are also POMs and you can't do an emergency supply for them. 2: False. Check carefully! It is not a legal requirement, but an ethical one. See service specification standard number 15. The question is not without a fault however – if you miss the implication of the word 'legal' and decide it's true, the next bit is easy – it cannot be an explanation of statement 1. You might have thought the skill is evaluation/synthesis, but as the answers are based on routine knowledge, it's just comprehension.
Q7	A	A	A	Statement 1 is true – as long as you sort out the unnecessary double negative. Remember the maths rule that two minuses make a plus. Statement 2 is also true – but the exact words are slightly different from those in the question. Any variation confuses candidates unfairly, and should be avoided. Hopefully that is the sort of point that would be picked up by the experienced pharmacist who acts as a reviewer of the questions. If it did get through, and a lot of candidates answered it incorrectly because that is not the exact wording in the Medicines Act, then the statistical analysis on an easy question that a large percentage would be expected to get right, would reveal the difficulty. Also note that the 'because' rule (AR4) used to decide whether two 'true' statements are connected works well in this example.

Table 4.3 Previously issued sample questions: a different analysis
Skills being tested K = knowledge C = comprehension A = application E = analysis/evaluation
Level of difficulty H = hard A = average E = easy

Question number	Open- or Closed-book	Multiple choice question style	Skill/s which is/are assessed	Level of difficulty	Answer code	Reason for choice of answer, including any 'implication' points made earlier that apply
Q1	open	SC	K	E	B	It's so unusual that it's remembered, PLUS SC2 – mixture of generic and brand names.
Q2	open	SC	C, K	E	D	Never mind about the ones you've never heard of, you don't sell aspirin for under-12s – think about it!
Q3	open	SC	A	A	D	The only one you are likely to have heard of is Dulco-lax – bisacodyl.
Q4	closed	SC	K, C	E	B	By elimination, because you know the others are wrong, even if you don't know about Daktarin (miconazole) oral gel.
Q5	open	SC	E, C	A	C	There's quite a lot to do, but as long as you're careful with the numbers of each preparation, there shouldn't be any problems.
Q6	open	SC	A	H	C	They've all got to be looked up – do it alphabetically to save time.
Q7	closed	SC	K	H	D	If you really don't have a clue, the only way is to guess – but there's no point in returning later.
Q8	closed	SC	K	E	B	As above.
Q9	closed	SC	A	A	A	A question where, if it's closed-book, you might well be struggling to find an answer. Open-book, and it's easy – the requirement is for the date of birth, as long as you see the word 'not'.
Q10	open	MC	C	H	B	A crafty question, if you don't see the word 'alone'. The answer is that 1 and 2 are correct, which is an allowable combination PLUS MC1.

Table 4.3 (continued)

Question number	Open- or Closed-book	Multiple choice question style	Skill/s which is/are assessed	Level of difficulty	Answer code	Reason for choice of answer, including any 'implication' points made earlier that apply
Q11		MC	E	H	B	Not a very good question – it must surely encourage guessing – and what are the definitions to do with practice anyway? Some data to interpret would surely be more in keeping with the ethos of practice-based questions. An educated guess – number 3 refers to 'biexponential' decay – but 'bi' means two, so surely that can't be right! Also then you can't have 2 alone (MC2), so the answer must be B – the right answer, but possibly for the wrong reason.
Q12		MC	C, E	A	A	In a well-known multiple, a pharmacy manager is a specific job title; the question would be fairer if it referred to the 'manager of a pharmacy'.

Table 4.4 Answers and explanations of 'demonstrating pitfalls' multiple choice questions
Skills being tested K = knowledge C = comprehension A = application E = analysis/evaluation
Level of difficulty H = hard A = average E = easy

Demonstrating pitfalls question number	Open- or Closed-book	Multiple choice question style	Skill/s which is/are assessed	Level of difficulty	Answer code	Reason for choice of answer, including any 'implication' points made earlier that apply
Q1		AR	K	H	B	Lots to do for statement 1; convert the concentration to a percentage (2%), then check against the limitations for undivided preparations of codeine in the Medicines, Ethics and Practice guide. As it's >1.5% but <2.5%, it's classified as a CD Inv POM/Schedule 5 drug. Statement 2 is also true, but it does not explain 1, but repeats it. PLUS AR5.
Q2		AR	K	H	C (E without bits in brackets)	1. Without the information in the brackets, anyone who has used WWHAM will soon recognise that 'safely' has clinical implications, such as 'are the side-effects likely to be a problem' – so the answer would be false. But the question writer thinks of 'safe' in the legal sense – which is the reason for all the information about the football. See the beginning of the BNF about banned substances – to which the legal answer is true, which is what the writer intended to test. 2. Again, the answer has to be false, as hypertensive patients can use topical preparations. The use of the word systemic changes the whole focus of a perfectly appropriate question.
Q3		AR	A	A	B	The two statements are checking the understanding of the difference between 'personal control' and supervision, respectively. Although they are both true, statement 2 is not explaining number 1.
Q4		AR	E	H	B	Both statements can only be answered correctly if the student has not only read the relevant section in a recommended, not essential, text but has also evaluated it. As the book is now out of date, the question should be removed by the reviewers.

5

Questions and answers

5.1   Introduction

In the previous chapters, many aspects of learning during the preregistration year have been considered in order to try and help preregistration trainees meet the different challenges presented. However, for most graduates, the predominant concern during the year is passing the exam. Often, quite rightly, they feel that they can cope with gathering evidence, reaching the performance standards and even preparing and revising for themselves, but what they 'really, really want' is practice at doing exam questions to give them confidence. Well, here is a selection, together with a few notes of caution to read first:

- The questions that follow are not meant to be representative of a complete paper, or even half a paper, much less a whole exam – instead, they are an assortment of items set using the four MCQ styles.
- Questions are presented as open-book (Paper 2) followed by closed-book (Paper 1) examples.
- Each question has been classified according to the perceived difficulty and skill assessed, which are given with the answer codes, reasons and explanations on pp. 183–195.
- The above classifications, or question styles, are not meant to be representative of the relative numbers that might be set in the registration exam.
- Another very important point – the coverage of the syllabus content. Some topics have been included earlier, in the examples of questions to illustrate particular points, and there has also been a whole chapter dealing with calculations.
- The author has therefore tried to present questions from as many parts of the syllabus as possible, with the constraint that

questions are normally set by experts in the field. Consequently, some important areas are under-represented, and others only included at a somewhat basic level. It is also no doubt apparent that some (absolutely vital) sections of the syllabus are covered more than once; remember that just because a topic is listed in the syllabus, it doesn't mean that they all have equal importance and equal numbers of questions will be set on each.

● Every effort has been made to base the questions on practice-orientated scenarios and make them problem-solving, in order to test the skills of analysis and evaluation. Another aim has been to encourage preregistration trainees to use the reference sources a lot, in order to ensure that they are familiar with the contents. As a consequence there are far fewer Style 1 questions than normal, which tend to assess only one aspect of the syllabus and its aims.

● Some questions have been set on topics that are new to the syllabus and for which no sample questions had been issued at the time of writing. The intention is to provide some guidance as to the type of questions that might be set, although it is acknowledged that some will be found to be difficult.

● Hopefully the questions will be found to be demanding and useful as preparation and revision exercises, although it is acknowledged that in some respects they may not be representative of examples found on the papers.

● For each paper, the questions are split into groups according to question style and syllabus section. A summary of directions is given the *first* time each style is used. For the full instructions and explanations of the four different MCQ styles, refer to pp. 129–134.

● A final very important point – whilst every effort has been made to produce questions that meet the standards to which the writers work, the items have not been subjected to the rigorous process of review and refinement which happens to items that are accepted for the item bank.

5.2 Questions for open-book paper

5.2.1 Syllabus 1.11.a

Style 2

Each group of questions below consists of five lettered options followed by a list of numbered questions. For each numbered question select the one lettered option which is most closely related to it. Each lettered option may be used once, more than once, or not at all.

Questions 1–4 are about the drugs morphine and pholcodine, which are both examples of drugs that can fall into different legal categories depending on the amount of the active ingredient present. For the preparations of these drugs, select the appropriate answer from the possibilities given to complete the sentence.

A   0.2% w/v of base

B   0.02% w/v of base

C   0.3% w/v of base

D   2.5% w/v of base

E   1.5% w/v of base

Q1   Pholcodine Linctus BP is classified as a CD Inv P Medicine; it must contain less than . . .

Q2   Kaolin and Morphine Mixture BP is classified as a CD Inv P Medicine; it must contain less than . . .

Q3   Oramorph Concentrated Solution is classified as a CD POM; it must contain more than . . .

Q4   Oramorph Solution is classified as a CD Inv POM Medicine; it must contain less than . . .

5.2.2 Syllabus 1.11.b

For scenarios 5–7, decide, from the information given, which of the lettered codes best describes the legal situation.

A   Lack of personal control

B   Lack of supervision

C   There is a possibility that an offence against other legislation relevant to pharmacy has been committed

D   There is no breach of the law

E   There is a lack of personal control, supervision and possibly a breach of other legislation

Q5   A pharmacist wishes to attend the funeral service of his mother-in-law but cannot find a locum to take his place for the three hours he will need to be away from the shop. He notifies the local Health Authority that the shop will not be able to dispense NHS prescriptions for that time, but that the shop will be open for the sale of GSL medicines. The assistants will be told not to sell P medicines but to direct all customers to another local pharmacy.

Q6   The local police force enter the shop just as the local drug misusers are due for their instalments under the NHS arrangements. An unexploded bomb has been uncovered by workmen nearby, and the police want you to evacuate the shop at once. You decide to send the counter assistants home but need the dispensers to stay until the prescriptions, which have all been dispensed and checked, have been handed out. You leave the dispensers to give out the prescriptions while going with the police officers to remove oxygen cylinders to a safer storage area.

Q7   The pharmacy is very quiet and the pharmacist decides to do some paperwork in the office upstairs for the last half-hour until closing time. The counter staff are told to phone him if anyone asks for his advice, or wants a prescription doing, but they can continue to sell all medicines using the normal protocol.

5.2.3 Syllabus 1.11.a

Style 3

Directions summarised				
A 1, 2, 3	B 1, 2 only	C 2, 3 only	D 1 only	E 3 only

Q8 Some substances are so poisonous that even the controls on S1 poisons are insufficient; extra legal restrictions are placed on the substances before they can be sold, except for which of the following situations:

1 ☐ When sold for export

2 ☐ When sold for the purposes of research or chemical analysis

3 ☐ When sold by way of wholesale dealing

Style 4

Directions summarised	First statement	Second statement	
A	True	True	2nd statement is a correct explanation of the 1st
B	True	True	2nd statement is NOT a correct explanation of the 1st
C	True	False	
D	False	True	
E	False	False	

For questions 9–12, refer to the following 'prescription':

Town and Country Veterinary Group
The Gables
Anytown

For 'Rover'
c/o Mrs D. Norton
The Common
Anytown

Please Supply 1 × 10 mL Bottle Pilocarpine 1% Eye Drops
Instil 2 Drops Tds

For Animal Treatment Only
This treatment is For an Animal under my Care

Signed by a veterinary practitioner whose signature is recognised as genuine.

Name of the veterinary practitioner and qualifications.

	Statement 1	Statement 2
Q9	The above prescription is legal	It has the statement 'For Animal Treatment Only' on the prescription as a legal requirement
Q10	If a dispensed label for the above preparation was produced, it would need the name of the animal as a legal requirement on it	Dispensed labels for human and animal use are exactly the same, except for the addition of the name of the animal
Q11	The label for the above prescription would need the name of the owner as a legal requirement	Another additional requirement on a veterinary label is the words 'For Animal Treatment Only'
Q12	The above prescription is not legal	It is missing the date

Questions 13–17 refer to the scenario that follows:

If a professional person who is authorised to possess and supply a Controlled Drug (CD) wants to obtain supplies, that would be a wholesale supply, and is made on a requisition. Decide whether the following situations concerning such supplies are true or false.

	Statement 1	Statement 2
Q13	Before any wholesale supply can be made, the requisition has to be given to the pharmacist so that they can check it is legally correct and complete any necessary paperwork	The record in the CD register must be made at the time it is supplied – before it has left the shop
Q14	If a record of the wholesale supply is made in the CD register, it is not legally necessary to enter it in the Prescription Only Register (POR) too	If a record is kept in the POR, then there is no need to keep the requisition
Q15	The pharmacist can order supplies of CDs by telephone but all other professionals who are authorised to possess them need to submit an order in writing	The supply can only be made directly to the person that requests it
Q16	If you only supply five diamorphine injections to a doctor for her to use on her patients, the quantity is so small it makes it a retail supply	If a person who was unknown to you said that they were a doctor and needed some diamorphine injections to carry in their bag for use on visits, you *could* supply them
Q17	If you supply large quantities of codeine powder to a university for their research activities, it is a wholesale supply and you would probably need a wholesale dealer's licence	The 'drugs squad' officer can inspect your CD register and question or investigate any unusual supplies you make or receive

5.2.4 Syllabus 1.11a Sale and supply of medicines

Questions 18 and 19 concern the supply of Industrial Methylated Spirits (IMS).

Q18 Which of the following statements is/are true?

1 ☐ If a pharmacist wants to stock IMS for medicinal purposes, he has to obtain permission in writing by sending the appropriate form to the national headquarters of the Customs and Excise

2 ☐ Records must be kept of all supplies from the pharmacy of IMS; these must be kept for two years

3 ☐ The letter of authority from the Customs and Excise will specify

the exact conditions under which the pharmacist is permitted to keep IMS

Q19 Which of the following statements is/are true?

1 ☐ If a supply of IMS is made to a local medical practitioner, such as a nurse, the amount must not exceed 3 litres

2 ☐ If an athlete wishes to buy some surgical spirit in Edinburgh to rub on his feet before a marathon race, he must sign the Prescription Only Register; he does not need to do this if he wishes to make the same purchase locally before running in the London marathon

3 ☐ If the athlete in Statement 2 above wishes to make the purchase, he would have to go to a pharmacy in both instances

5.2.5 Syllabus 1.1.a The RPSGB Code of Ethics and (b) Clinical Governance

Style 2

A The personal responsibility of the pharmacist on duty

B A personal accountability of the pharmacist on duty

C A preregistration tutor's responsibility

D A superintendent's responsibility

E A superintendent's accountability

For questions 20–25, choose from the answers A to E the one that best fits accountability and/or responsibility for the scenario described.

Q20 An elderly, slightly confused patient is prescribed MST tablets. She normally has all her weekly medication dispensed (by a pharmacist working for a small chain of pharmacies) in a compliance aid, which the doctor wants to continue, as she lives on her own.

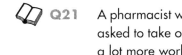 **Q21** A pharmacist working for a large chain of pharmacies has recently been asked to take on the dispensing for a new residential home; it will mean a lot more work to assemble the prescriptions each month but there are many opportunities for medicines management activities. He thinks that a new PMR system might need to be installed to ensure that the requirements of the Data Protection Act can be adhered to; his area manager, who is not a pharmacist, does not agree.

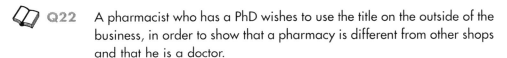 **Q22** A pharmacist who has a PhD wishes to use the title on the outside of the business, in order to show that a pharmacy is different from other shops and that he is a doctor.

Q23 The local police force come into the shop and identify themselves. They are investigating suspicious deaths which involve the use of sodium amytal. They want you to search your records and tell them the names of everyone who has had it prescribed to them in the last year.

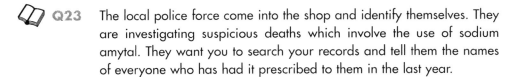 **Q24** A child of eight calls to collect her grandmother's antibiotic capsules. A neighbour left the prescription as the old lady is ill in bed.

Q25 A new preregistration trainee, who was previously employed by one organisation, starts work for another multiple pharmacy. She does not tell the pharmacist on duty when she sells a packet of Pharmacy Only throat sweets. When questioned, she says that in her previous company, the training and the protocol that was in use meant that she did not have to. The customer complains that the product is unsuitable and that no questions were asked when it was sold.

Style 3

Questions 26–30 refer to the three advertisements:

Day and Night Pharmacy	Day and Night Pharmacy	Day and Night Pharmacy
George Day takes pleasure in announcing that his business will be transferred to his new pharmacy at 109 Night Road Anytown Telephone 01234 567 890	George Day takes pleasure in announcing that his business will be transferred to his new pharmacy at 109 Night Road Anytown Telephone 01234 567 890	George Day takes pleasure in announcing that his business will be transferred to his new pharmacy at 109 Night Road Anytown Telephone 01234 567 890
Hours of business Monday to Saturday 9.00 a.m. to 6 p.m. Oxygen delivery Repeat Prescription Collection Service Aromatherapy and Reflexology a speciality. We guarantee a quick and accurate service!! 10% Discount given to all new customers!!	Hours of business Monday to Saturday 9.00 a.m. to 6 p.m. Oxygen delivery Repeat Prescription Collection Service Pregnancy Testing Your local chemist, offering a faster service	Pharmacy Hours of business Monday to Saturday 9.00 a.m. to 6 p.m. Oxygen delivery Nursing Home Service Free Health Care Advice Pregnancy Testing by specially trained staff
Advertisement 1	Advertisement 2	Advertisement 3

Study the advertisements carefully and then answer questions 26–30 by comparing the statement about the advertisement and the following statements:

1 The statement is true for advertisement 1
2 The statement is true for advertisement 2
3 The statement is true for advertisement 3

Q26 Statement: The services mentioned in the advertisement are all core services that would be offered from every pharmacy and are therefore subject to the controls of Service Specification (SS) 1 of the Code of Ethics.

Q27 Statement: The wording of the advertisement is acceptable even though some restricted titles are used.

Q28 Statement: It is unacceptable to imply that the dispensing service or any other professional service offered is superior to that of other pharmacists. The advertisement is guilty of this misdemeanour.

 Q29 Statement: It is unacceptable to offer an inducement to the public in relation to professional services. The advertisement does not comply with the Medicines (Advertising) Regulations in this respect.

 Q30 Statement: If the highlighted information was deleted from the advertisement, it would fulfil SS 1 of the Code of Ethics.

Style 4

Questions 31–34 concern the Code of Ethics and Practice Advice.

	Statement 1	Statement 2
Q31	The Practice Guidance is additional Information to that in the Code of Ethics and the Standards or Service Specifications	The Practice Guidance is issued by the Council of the RPSGB and is intended to give additional advice on every Service Specification
Q32	The practice guidance consists of statements about the aims, provision, delivery, evaluation and training for a professional service	The practice guidance is intended to help meet the professional requirements of a service specification
Q33	Pharmacists can apply for a customs and excise licence to sell tonic wine	Pharmacists who sell alcohol must not contribute to the problems that it can cause by promoting its use or by selling a product that could mask its use
Q34	A pharmacist could use his or her mobile phone to contact a patient whose number is ex-directory in an emergency under the scheme set up with BT in 1998	A pharmacist who has dispensed some warfarin tablets instead of the ones that were intended would need to get in touch with the patient as a matter of life or death

Style 1

 Q35 Select the most appropriate answer from the statements concerning a standard operating procedure for the sale of Pharmacy Medicines

A ☐ It is designed to provide an answer in every instance where an over the counter medication is requested

B ☐ It is to be followed by all the staff and locum pharmacists without exception

C ☐ It is to give minimal guidance – it's then up to the staff to interpret the request and how to deal with it

D ☐ A standard operating procedure must be written and on display

E ☐ It is to ensure that a request for a named medication is turned into a situation where advice can be offered

5.2.6 Syllabus 2.1.b The action and uses of drugs

Style 2

Questions 36–39 refer to preparations of the following non-steroidal anti-inflammatory drugs (NSAIDs):

A Mefenamic acid
B Diclofenac
C Ketoprofen
D Meloxicam
E Ibuprofen

Q36 The maximum daily dose by any route is 150 mg.

Q37 A prescription for two capsules to be taken three times a day represents the maximum daily dose.

Q38 A preparation is available in the form of modified-release capsules containing white pellets, to be taken once daily.

Q39 The drug is available in a long acting preparation, with a recommended dose of two tablets to be taken in the early evening.

Questions 40–42 refer to drugs that act on the gastro-intestinal system. Choose the most appropriate one.

A   Omeprazole
B   Lansoprazole
C   Nizatidine
D   Cimetidine
E   Gaviscon

Q40   A child of eight develops severe ulcerating reflux oesophagitis; the paediatric consultant initiates a course of . . .

Q41   An asthma sufferer has been taking theophylline for many years; he has now developed a gastric ulcer. His doctor wishes to keep prescribing costs as low as possible but still offer a clinically effective drug as first line treatment.

Q42   An obese elderly lady suffers with heartburn. She is advised to follow a low-fat diet and to give up smoking. She is prescribed a medication to help with the symptoms until the underlying cause can be diagnosed.

Questions 43–45 refer to drugs that act on the cardiovascular system. Choose the most appropriate one to complete the sentence.

A   Bendroflumethiazide (bendrofluazide) 2.5 mg
B   Bendroflumethiazide (bendrofluazide) 5 mg
C   Atenolol 50 mg
D   Atenolol 100 mg
E   Indapamide

Q43   A 60-year-old lady with a tendency to 'wheeziness' is found to have slightly raised blood pressure when she is assessed after a stroke; she is prescribed . . .

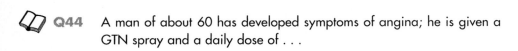 **Q44** A man of about 60 has developed symptoms of angina; he is given a GTN spray and a daily dose of . . .

Q45 A lady who has Type 2 diabetes needs a drug to control hypertension; she is otherwise healthy. The GP chooses . . .

Questions 46–47 and 48–49 refer to drugs that act on the central nervous system. Choose the most appropriate to complete the sentence.

A   Nitrazepam 2.5 mg
B   Nitrazepam 5 mg
C   Temazepam 20 mg
D   Zopiclone 3.75 mg
E   Zopiclone 7.5 mg

Q46 An elderly lady is very upset following the death of her friend; she is prescribed a short course of . . . to help her sleep.

Q47 A gentleman in his 50s sees his doctor about his acute anxiety state. He has been told to close his firm by the receivers and he is very worried about his employees. He is prescribed . . . and warned about the possible effects on his ability to drive.

A   Amitriptyline
B   Dosulepin (dothiepin)
C   Citalopram
D   Fluoxetine
E   Paroxetine

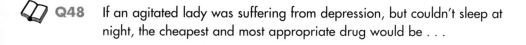 **Q48** If an agitated lady was suffering from depression, but couldn't sleep at night, the cheapest and most appropriate drug would be . . .

Q49 For a depressed lady who did not need sedating, . . . would be chosen, especially as she is prone to panic attacks.

Questions 50–53 refer to drugs that act on the musculoskeletal and joint systems. Choose the most appropriate one/s.

A   Paracetamol
B   Paracetamol and codeine
C   Ibuprofen tablets
D   Naproxen tablets
E   Diclofenac tablets SR

 Q50 An asthmatic lady has been diagnosed as having spondylitis. She cannot move very much and gets easily constipated. She is prescribed . . . to help with the pain.

 Q51 A housebound elderly man cannot get out of bed in the morning, as his joints are so stiff. Once moving, he can cope quite well with assistance from carers.

 Q52 An athlete has 'pulled a muscle'. He has applied an ice pack and rested, but is still in pain. He is prescribed the most cost effective remedy for the condition.

 Q53 An overweight businessman has an acute attack of gout; the doctor suggests trying one of the above, in the hope that it will act fairly quickly.

5.2.7 Syllabus 2.11c Formulation and preparation

	Statement 1	Statement 2
Q54	A mixture of solid drugs to be taken internally is supplied as dry powder, which is mixed in water before being taken. An example is Magnesium Trisilicate Oral Powder Compound BP	A possible reason for supplying a powder in bulk is to reduce the inconvenience for the patient of carrying large bottles of medicine
Q55	An individual powder is a possible dosage form for a child who is prescribed a potent drug that is not available in the dose requested	An individual wrapped powder formulation of a lipid soluble drug could be used to administer the drug quickly for maximum absorption orally

5.3 Questions for closed-book paper

5.3.1 Syllabus 1.11a

Style 2

For the following questions, 56–60, you will need to refer to Table 5.1. Choose the lettered option that exactly fits the legal classification given in the question.

Q56 CD Inv P

Q57 CD Anab POM

Q58 CD Benz POM

Q59 CD No Register POM

Q60 CD POM

Table 5.1

Specific requirement	A	B	C	D	E
Do pharmacists have authority to possess and supply?	✓	✓	✓	✓	✓
Is a licence needed to import/export as wholesaler?	✓	✗	✓	✗	✓
Must generally be kept in CD cupboard?	✗	✗	✗	✗	✓
Does anyone need to supervise their destruction?	✗	✗	✗	✗	✓
Is a requisition needed for a wholesale supply?	✗	✗	✓	✗	✓
Is it possible for them to be available to the public for sale?	✗	✗	✗	✓	✗

Key: ✓ = Where the answer to the question about whether or not a legal requirement needs to be fulfilled for examples of preparations in that classification is yes.
✗ = Where the answer to the question about whether or not a specific requirement needs to be fulfilled is no.

For the following questions, 61–65, you will need to refer to Table 5.2. For each of the CD classifications given, choose the lettered code that matches the prescription requirements described.

Q61   CD Inv P

Q62   CD Inv POM

Q63   CD Benz POM

Q64   CD No Register POM

Q65   CD POM

Table 5.2

	A	B	C	D	E
Do all details except doctor's name and address need to be handwritten?	✓	✗	✓	✗	✗
Does the quantity in words and figures have to be on?	✓	✗	✓	✗	✗
Does the 'Form' need to be included?	✓	✗	✓	✗	✗
Does a record need to be made in the CD register?	✗	✗	✓	✗	✗
Can a private prescription be returned to the customer, even if no repeats are indicated?	✗	✗	✗	✓	✗
Do the dose and frequency need to be stated?	✓	✗	✓	✗	✗
Is it only valid for 13 weeks?	✓	✗	✓	✗	✗
Does the invoice have to be kept for two years?	✓	✓	✗	✓	✗

Key: ✓ = Where the answer to the question about whether or not a legal requirement needs to be fulfilled (for examples of preparations in that classification) is yes.
✗ = Where the answer to the question is no.

For the following questions, 66–69, you will need to refer to Table 5.3. For each of the preparations given, choose the lettered code that matches the prescription requirements described.

(Do them as open-book if you don't know the legal classification of each.)

 Q66 Temazepam tablets 10 mg on an NHS prescription.

Q67   Temgesic tablets 200 mcg on an NHS prescription.

 Q68   Dexamethasone tablets 2 mg on an NHS prescription.

 Q69   Nitrazepam tablets 5 mg on a private prescription.

Table 5.3

	A	B	C	D	E
Patient's name and address must be handwritten by the prescriber	✓	✓	✗	✗	✗
Prescription must be dated by the prescriber	✓	✓	✗	✗	✗
Strength must be stated as a legal requirement	✗	✓	✗	✗	✗
An emergency supply at the request of a doctor can be made	✗	✗	✗	✓	✓
No repeats allowed	✓	✓	✓	✓	✗
Product must be stored in the CD cupboard	✓	✓	✓	✗	✗

Key: ✓ = Where the requirement in the statement must be complied with.
✗ = Where the requirement is not a legal necessity.

Style 3

For questions 70–72, decide which of the details, below, are legally needed on private prescriptions in the following situations.

1   Name and address of patient/carer/owner
2   Name and address of doctor
3   Age of patient

Q70 A prescription for bendroflumethiazide (bendrofluazide) for a dog.

 Q71 A prescription for amoxicillin for a child of five.

 Q72 A prescription for pethidine for a man of 56.

5.3.2 Syllabus 1.11d, e, f

Style 2

For questions 73 and 74 that follow, choose from the following answers:

A   The Control of Substances Hazardous to Health (COSHH) Regulations

B   The Controlled Waste Regulations 1992

C   The Environmental Protection Act 1990

D   The Collection and Disposal of Waste Regulations 1988

E   The Producer Responsibility Obligations (Packaging Waste) 1997

 Q73 Under which of the above Acts can a householder arrange disposal of 'clinical' waste, such as used insulin syringes?

 Q74 Under which of the above Acts might a community pharmacist have a responsibility for recycling the cardboard containers in which the Controlled Drugs they receive are packed?

Style 3

 Q75 Which of the following statements is/are true about the Data Protection Act 1998?

1   Personal data shall not be processed unless certain conditions are met

2   Personal date means any information by which a living individual can be identified

3   The Data Protection Act has now been extended to cover paper records as well as computerised ones.

Style 4

Questions 76–78 refer to the Trade Descriptions Act.

	Statement 1	Statement 2
Q76	The Trade Descriptions Act of 1968 provides controls against misleading the public when describing goods and services	Under the Act, a trade has a very narrow meaning and excludes businesses and professions
Q77	If a customer makes a specific request, and the supplier cannot reasonably check that the request has been fulfilled, then the supplier can plead that they relied on the information supplied which was inadequate	An offence is committed under the Act if the statement was known to be false, or not enough care was taken to establish its accuracy
Q78	A trade description includes reference to the quantity, size, composition, and production method of the goods	It is not necessary to declare the country of origin of a medicine, although it is for other goods

5.3.3   Syllabus 1.11a, b Sale and supply of (OTC) medicines and Code of Ethics

Style 2

Q79   Which one of the following OTC preparations is the most likely to be the subject of regular purchases that may necessitate further questioning?

A   ☐ Nylax tablets
B   ☐ Milk of magnesia tablets
C   ☐ Lactulose syrup
D   ☐ Fybogel sachets
E   ☐ Syrup of figs

Q80 Which one of the following OTC preparations is the most likely to be the subject of regular purchases that may necessitate further questioning?

A ☐ Piriton tablets
B ☐ Stugeron tablets
C ☐ Dramamine tablets
D ☐ Benadryl allery relief
E ☐ Clarityn syrup

For question numbers 81–84, choose from:

A   The action that was taken was not ethical – either it does not conform to or it contradicts the guidance given by the RPSGB in the Code of Ethics

B   The action that was taken was not legal or ethical – it does not conform to the provisions of the Medicines Act or the Code of Ethics

C   A supply was made that was legal and ethical, as described above

D   An ethical consideration was made, but there was a breach of the Medicines Act

E   An ethical consideration was made; there was no breach of the Medicines Act

Q81 A pharmacist receives a prescription for a medication for hypertension from an American customer; he decides to dispense it as it is late on a Saturday and the customer assures him that he must have the drug as he has run out.

Q82 The medicines counter assistant asks you to supervise the sale of six large packs (each containing 32 tablets) of paracetamol 500 mg tablets. The customer is going abroad for an extended stay and needs them for a painful medical condition; his doctor cannot write an NHS prescription because they are for treatment outside the UK, so you supply them.

Q83 A pharmacy seems to be selling a lot more Feminax tablets than normal.

The pharmacist decides to make all sales himself in order to monitor the situation. When questioned, one purchaser says she buys them for the other ladies in the office where she works. The pharmacist supplies her with two packets on this occasion, but decides to discuss the situation with other pharmacists in the area.

 Q84 A pharmacist is taken ill soon after arriving at work and decides to go home, leaving the shop open. He cannot get a locum pharmacist to come until the next day, so he instructs his staff to send any prescriptions to the pharmacy down the road; they cannot give out any completed prescriptions, as there are some CDs amongst them for a patient who is terminally ill. They must not sell P medicines in his absence either.

5.3.4 **Syllabus 2.1d Differentiating between minor illness and more serious disease**

Style 2

For questions 85–86, choose from the following symptoms of childhood feverish illnesses:

A   Swollen lymph nodes on back of neck
B   Pink rash that blanches with pressure
C   Rash that lasts several days
D   Feeling ill before the rash appears
E   Red spots with small white centres on the inside of the cheeks

 Q85 The symptom that is unique to measles.

 Q86 The symptom that is much more likely to be an indication of German measles (Rubella) than measles.

Questions 87–90: For the following scenarios, the deciding factor concerning the treatment recommended is:

A   Duration of symptoms

B   Severity of symptoms

C   Person suffering from the symptoms

D   Additional factors

E   What the patient/carer thinks

Q87   Mrs G comes in with her youngest child, baby Matthew, who is eight weeks old. The previous evening he had several dirty nappies but was feeding normally, so she was not unduly worried about him. However since this morning he has refused two feeds and is very hot. As he is too young to be sold Diorylate, you suggest increasing his intake of fluids with drinks of boiled water and referral to the GP today.

Q88   Ms G is normally a regular customer for her 'pill' prescription; when you see her in the shop you realise that she hasn't been collecting it recently. She describes a pain low down in her side that she has had for 'a few days'. Although she hasn't been sick, she feels queasy and has not been eating very much. She thinks she may have a temperature and wants to know if she can have some ibuprofen tablets, as its obviously the 'flu that is going round.

Q89   Mr J is a frequent visitor to your pharmacy for films which he takes on his many business trips abroad; his firm frequently send him to un-developed countries to sell water purifying equipment. He has had diarrhoea since returning from his latest trip last week. He has tried Imodium and found them reasonably effective, but wonders if there is anything better. You suggest he really should see his GP.

Q90   Mrs K is very concerned about her only daughter, who is 12 and beginning to get a few 'teenage spots' on her face; she thinks they are due to 'overheated blood' and asks for some sulphur tablets, just like she used to take, to 'clear the blood'. You spend some time reassuring both mother and daughter that the spots are not catching, and sell appropriate skin preparations.

For questions 91–94, choose from:

A   Go to the doctor as soon as possible

B   Go to the Accident and Emergency department of the nearest hospital as a matter of urgency

C   Sell an appropriate remedy

D   Recommend the use of a 'home remedy' such as an ice pack or hot water bottle

E   Go to the GP in two or three days if the condition does not improve

Q91   An elderly lady requests a bottle of eye drops; her eyes are red and inflamed. She has previously seen the doctor for the condition, who prescribed Chloromycetin drops, which she used every two hours for five days. The condition got a little better at first, but is now getting worse again.

Q92   An elderly lady asks to see the pharmacist. Since she woke up this morning, she has had what she can only describe as a 'bubble' in one eye. She cannot see very well in it, and it hurts a bit. It doesn't appear to be red or inflamed.

Q93   It is a hot sunny day in May; a lady of about 35 wants something to stop the irritation in her eyes. They are very red and inflamed, but there are no other signs of infection. She is also sneezing frequently. She has not yet tried anything, but takes the oral contraceptive pill.

Q94   A gentleman dressed in football kit limps into the pharmacy. He has received an injury to his ankle. The coach at the club applied some 'smelly stuff' that made it go very red, and his doctor told him to take ibuprofen tablets, which he is doing. He wants to know if there is anything else that he can do to get himself fit enough for the big match next week.

Style 3

Q95 A wasp in your shop has stung a child of six. You calm the child and the mother and apply a well-known remedy containing a local anaesthetic, and give instructions to seek medical advice if:

1 There is difficulty breathing
2 The area is still slightly red after four hours
3 There is further pain in the immediate area of the sting

For questions 96–98 choose from:

1 Extra fluids
2 Dioralyte sachets
3 Loperamide in a suitable dose

Q96 A child of seven complains of stomach cramps and occasional diarrhoea. In addition to suggesting that he does not eat for 24 hours, which of the above do you recommend?

Q97 A lady of about 75 complains of a worsening of the diarrhoea she gets, which is associated with diverticular disease. She has a routine appointment with her doctor tomorrow; she expects he will also increase the dose of codeine which she takes continually. Can you recommend anything else in the meantime?

Q98 A couple in their 30s have just returned from a wonderful holiday backpacking in India. Unfortunately, they have both developed diarrhoea since their return; neither of them is really ill – but it's very inconvenient now they are back at work. They know about the diseases that they might have picked up, and will see their GP if their symptoms worsen. Can they have anything to try and stop it?

5.3.5   Syllabus 2.1h Counselling requirements

Style 2

For questions 99–101 choose from:

A   A middle aged lady with a repeat prescription for bendroflumethi-azide (bendrofluazide)

B   A young mother who is very anxious to get home to her family; she is collecting a repeat prescription for her oral contraceptive tablets.

C   A teenager who is collecting an inhaler for her mother who does not speak English. She has had the medication before.

D   A smartly dressed lady who is rattling her car keys impatiently. She is collecting a new prescription for a type of HRT that has only recently come onto the market.

E   A carer who is collecting the tablets in compliance aids for several of her elderly residents, as she does every week.

Q99   Which one of the above would you *always* want to counsel about their medication?

Q100   Which one of the above would you try to counsel at a home visit rather than in the shop?

Q101   Which one of the above is generally most likely to need counselling?

5.3.6   Syllabus 2.1e

Style 2

Questions 102–107: For each of the drugs listed below, select, from the possible answers A–E, the *most* likely Adverse Drug Reaction:

A   Gingival hyperplasia

B   Dry mouth

C   Nausea and vomiting

D   Diarrhoea

E   Constipation

Q102 Clindamycin.

Q103 Digoxin.

Q104 Fluoxetine.

Q105 Sodium valproate.

Q106 Codeine.

Q107 Lisinopril.

5.3.7   Syllabus 2.1i Optimising patients' drug therapy

Style 2

For questions 108–110 choose from:

A   Tablet

B   Capsule

C   Suppository

D   Liquid

E   Sugar-free liquid

Q108 A four-year-old boy starts to have seizures; he is prescribed sodium valproate. The dose is gradually increased until his seizures are controlled. He is to remain on the medication for at least six months.

Q109 A patient is prescribed medication for her migraines; her first symptom is severe nausea, followed by vomiting and then the headache develops.

Q110 An adult customer complains of a very sore throat; she is having a great deal of difficulty eating. Her doctor decides that the cause is bacterial and gives her a course of penicillin.

Questions 111–113.

A   Penicillin V
B   Rifampicin
C   Erythromycin
D   Amoxicillin
E   Ciprofloxacin

Which of the above is the drug of choice in the prophylaxis of:

 Q111 Meningitis.

 Q112 An infection caused by dental procedures in patients who have a heart condition.

 Q113 Whooping cough.

For questions 114–117, choose from:

A   Vitamin A
B   Vitamin B$_{12}$
C   Vitamin C
D   Vitamin D
E   Folic acid

 Q114 A patient prescribed methotrexate is often also prescribed this.

 Q115 A patient prescribed a calcium supplement often needs this too.

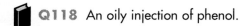 **Q116** This is only effective parenterally.

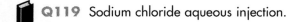 **Q117** All those planning to conceive should take this.

5.3.8 Syllabus 2.11.c

Style 3

For questions 118–120, which of the following is/are suitable methods of sterilising the products given:

1   Dry heat
2   Another method
3   Saturated steam

Q118 An oily injection of phenol.

Q119 Sodium chloride aqueous injection.

Q120 Sterile dressing packs.

5.4   Concluding remarks

There is not very much to add, except to emphasise a point made several times before – that the passing of the exam is only one condition for registration, and that these questions are not representative of an examination paper. However, using them as a revision tool, and trying to develop the skills that are necessary to pass the registration exam, will also help you in practice. Good luck in what will hopefully be the final stage in the process of achieving registration.

5.5   Answers and analysis of sample questions

5.5.1   Answers and explanations of sample questions

See Table 5.4 for answers and explanations

Table 5.4

Question number	Answer code	Reason
Open book		
Q1	E	For undivided preparations of pholcodine the ms to be a CD Inv P is 1.5% w/v.
Q2	B	For undivided preparations of morphine the ms to be a CD Inv P is 0.02% w/v.
Q3	A	For undivided preparations of morphine the ms to be a CD Inv POM is 0.2% w/v, so a stronger product must be CD POM.
Q4	A	As above.
Q5	A	The Medicines Act states that even to sell GSL medicines, a pharmacy must be under the personal control of a pharmacist, which is generally recognised as an absence of not more than one hour; there is no breach of supervision or other laws.
Q6	E	There are a lot of issues here; the health and safety of employees, supervision of dispensing – which means the handing out of completed prescriptions too, and he is probably not in personal control either.
Q7	B	As he is still on the premises, and has given instructions, he is still in personal control, but not in a position to intervene.
Q8	A	Easy – as long as you know where to look in the Medicines, Ethics and Practice guide.
Q9	E	Statement 1: False – for reason, see later. Statement 2: False – needs to be on the label, not the prescription.
Q10	E	Statement 1: False – name of owner a legal requirement. Statement 2: False – they also need the address where the animal is kept.
Q11	B	Statement 1: True. Statement 2: True but not the correct explanation.
Q12	A	Statement 1: True. Statement 2: True, and it's an explanation of statement 1.
Q13	E	Statement 1: False – a practitioner has 24 hours in which to supply the requisition; other persons requesting the CD must supply it in advance. Needless to say, the pharmacist would not supply the CD unless they were sure that the request was genuine, and that the legally necessary document would be forthcoming. Statement 2: False – entries must be made on the day of the supply, or on the following day; they must be chronological.

continued overleaf

Table 5.4 (*continued*)

Question number	Answer code	Reason
Q14	C	Statement 1: True. Statement 2: False; they must be kept for 2 years.
Q15	C	Statement 1: True. Statement 2: False – the person who is authorised to possess can send a third party to collect the CD; however, they need an authorisation, in writing, from the recipient if they are not automatically authorised to possess – as in the case of a delivery driver from the wholesalers for example.
Q16	D	Statement 1: False – the purchase for administration to another is one of the definitions of a wholesale supply. Statement 2: True – but of course you would need to establish a few facts first!
Q17	D	Statement 1: False – because the university are using the codeine themselves, it is still a retail sale. Remember there are very strict controls on the persons within the university that can be supplied, and that checks will be made of the CD register, especially if large quantities are involved. Statement 2: True – see Statement 1.
Q18	E	1. False – the pharmacist has to apply to the local office of Customs and Excise on the required form. 2. False – it is only the supplies 'other than on prescription' for which records have to be kept. 3. True – the conditions will vary from office to office, but will cover storage, use, labelling and supply.
Q19	D	1. True – the amount must not exceed 3 litres. It is also important to note that the term 'practitioner' has a different meaning to that in the Medicines Act, and includes nurses and chiropodists. 2. False – There used to be additional controls on the sale of 'meths' and surgical spirits in Scotland, which included the recording of such a sale, but the change in legislation applies to surgical spirits too. No entry is necessary. 3. False – The athlete *could* go to a pharmacist lawfully conducting a retail pharmacy business in Scotland or in England. However the additional sellers in Scotland are still authorised to sell spirits, although they no longer have to be registered.
Q20	A	So long as the pharmacist has checked with the doctor and assessed the risks against the possible benefits, and perhaps considered the alternatives, there must be at least joint accountability with the doctor. Also a clear need to consider their duty of care to the patient and her wishes too – she is probably adamant that she won't go into a home. The pharmacist is definitely responsible but probably not accountable in the event of a mishap.
Q21	E	This is a different situation, which obviously depends on what action is taken by the large chain. If the system was not updated and the law was broken,

Table 5.4   (*continued*)

Question number	Answer code	Reason
		then the superintendent is accountable for the failure to provide an adequate system.
Q22	B	Under the old Code, there was a specific restriction on using such titles. The new Code is much less prescriptive, and relies on the integrity of the pharmacist in such situations. Look at SS 1 regarding publicity – (a) refers to not exploiting the lack of knowledge of the public – so you will be in trouble if you are seen to do so – and therefore accountable for your actions.
Q23	B	It's not just a responsibility, you will be accountable to answer for your actions if do not make the proper checks with regard to C (b) as it is a personal responsibility to maintain confidentiality.
Q24	A	The use of the medicinal product and the necessary advice must be passed on, and the method of delivery must be safe. As no face to face contact will take place between the pharmacist and the patient – SS 4.1(i) – there must be no doubt that SS 8 (a) is fully considered. Your PR demands that you are responsible for the wellbeing and safety of all patients; you will need to consider the risks carefully as you will also be accountable for your actions in the event of anything going wrong that you could have foreseen. A phone call may well be an appropriate measure to explore if a safe delivery is possible, and to pass on advice. Your eventual decision may well depend on the medication, its packaging and the distance the child has to travel. Another example where keeping a record of what you did and why is very important, in case you have to prove that you carried out your duty of care to the best of your ability and how a competent pharmacist ought to have behaved in the same circumstances. SS 8 delivery (c) audit trail.
Q25	B	The pharmacy superintendent is ultimately responsible for the records which indicate which pharmacist is on duty at any time and as such is accountable for all the activities of non-pharmacists involved in the provision of pharmacy services. He or she is also accountable for the protocol, which may well state that a suitably qualified assistant may sell certain P medicines without intervention, so long as supervision is allowed for. It will often exclude certain products – recent POM to P changes, for example. The Superintendent is accountable for providing a protocol, and the pharmacist if it goes wrong or is not applied. A difficult situation that must be handled carefully by all concerned.
Q26	C	For advertisement 1: False. For advertisement 2: True. For advertisement 3: True. In the guidance on publicity and promotion (SS 1) which would of course include advertising, the introduction states that the SSs cover a range of services, and that some are core and some additional. In SS 12, which refers to complementary therapies, it implies that any pharmacists offering such services must have undergone extra training, so aromatherapy etc. is not a

continued overleaf

Table 5.4 (continued)

Question number	Answer code	Reason
		core service. It may still come within the additional ones however and be covered by SS 1 provision of health care advice, services to nursing homes and a repeat collection service, for example.
Q27	A	Advertisement 1: True. Advertisement 2: True Advertisement 3: True.
		Under the Medicines Act, certain titles such as 'pharmacist' and 'chemist' are restricted to pharmacists in order to protect the public. It would appear that when publicising the professional services available, it is acceptable to use the terms in order to inform the public that it is indeed a qualified health professional offering the services.
Q28	A	Advertisement 1: True. Advertisement 2: True. Advertisement 3: True.
		SS 1(b) clearly states that publicity for professional services must not disparage or make claims of superiority to the professional services offered by other pharmacists. Advertisement 1 describes its dispensing service as quick and accurate; advertisement 2 claims to offer a faster service, and advertisement 3 has 'specially trained staff' to carry out pregnancy testing. All of these advertisements therefore could be interpreted to imply that the service offered is superior to that in another pharmacy, thus contravening the advertising guidelines.
Q29	A	Advertisement 1: True. Advertisement 2: True Advertisement 3: True
		Let's look at the first part of the 'stem' first. SS1 gives advice to pharmacists and their responsibilities with regard to the promotion of their services. Advice is concerned with emphasising the special nature of medicines and not offering inducements that persuade someone to buy more than is needed, which is perceived to be unprofessional. In advertisement 1 a '10% discount is given to all new customers' is offered, which could be thought to contravene the advice; however, the advertisement does not make clear that the 10% discount applies to professional services. Perhaps the pharmacist did not intend the offer to extend to the professional side of the business, but did not realise the implications of the wording chosen in this context. In a similar manner, it is debatable whether the wording for advertisement 3 – offering 'free health care advice' – is acceptable, as every pharmacist does just that every day. The key is being aware of some guidance tucked away under general legal requirements in the Medicines, Ethics and Practice guide. The medicines advertising regulations apply to inducements offered to health professionals by drug manufacturers for example, not the public – so each statement is true, they do not conform.

Table 5.4   (*continued*)

Question number	Answer code	Reason
Q30	C	Advertisement 1: False Advertisement 2: True. Advertisement 3: True. With the last statement removed, both 2 and 3 are acceptable. They are reasonably dignified and would not bring the profession into disrepute or mislead the public, whilst at the same time informing them of the availability of professional services. Advertisement 1 still 'guarantees a quick and accurate service' – which cannot be accurate or honest.
Q31	C	Statement 1: True – see Medicines, Ethics and Practice guide Section 3. Statement 2: False – although the advice is issued by the Council of the RPSGB, it does not cover every SS.
Q32	A	Statement 1: True – see headings under each service. Statement 2: True – as clearly stated in the aims of each item of guidance, which is an explanation of why it contains aims etc., so code A.
Q33	B	Statement 1: True – it would be illegal to sell the wine without one. Statement 2: True – see SS 2 for the details; the statement is a separate point rather than an explanation.
Q34	A	Statement 1: True – see details of the scheme in section 3.4.6. of the miscellaneous practice guidance. It should be noted that the pharmacists could use a mobile phone, but the operator must be convinced that the call is made from the community pharmacy premises. Statement 2: True – no matter what the intended tablets were, if someone took warfarin instead, it could be fatal, which is precisely why the scheme exists.
Q35	E	This is the only description that can be acceptable within the spirit of the intentions for protocols, as described in the Medicines, Ethics and Practice guide.
Q36	B	For all these questions (36–39), very careful scrutiny of the BNF will reveal the answers. The intention is for you to practice the skill.
Q37	A	
Q38	C	
Q39	E	
Q40	A	Questions 40–53 are designed to test the ability to solve problems and to provide practice at searching for detailed information in the BNF, roughly according to the order of the categories. The answers are all there – make sure you look carefully at all the licensed indications.
Q41	C	
Q42	E	
Q43	A	
Q44	D	
Q45	E	
Q46	C	
Q47	C/E	
Q48	A	

continued overleaf

Table 5.4 (*continued*)

Question number	Answer code	Reason
Q49	C	
Q50	A	
Q51	E	
Q52	C	
Q53	D	
Q54	A	Statement 1: True – instructions in the BNF refer to Label 13. Statement 2: True – reasonable reason, so A.
Q55	C	Statement 1: True. Statement 2: False – most drugs that are formulated for rapid absorption are soluble in water; lipid soluble drugs are not soluble in water! Read *Pharmaceutical Practice* p. 161.
Closed book		
Q56	D	Questions 56–60 are examples of application – the information is known to all, it is just asked for in a novel manner.
Q57	A	
Q58	B	
Q59	C	
Q60	E	
Q61	D	Questions 61–65 are examples of application – the information is known to all, it is just asked for in a novel manner.
Q62	B	
Q63	E	
Q64	A	
Q65	C	
Q66	C	Again, Questions 66–69 are testing basic knowledge in a different manner – the problem-solving ability should be well developed by now.
Q67	B	
Q68	D	
Q69	E	
Q70	D	Basic legal requirements (Questions 70 and 71); remember that number 70 will need the name and address of the vet, not a doctor!
Q71	A	
Q72	B	No age needed as not under 12.
Q73	D	Under the Collection and Disposal of Waste Regulations 1988, a householder can dispose of such waste, designated 'clinical' waste, and the local authority has a duty to collect it (although they may charge a fee).
Q74	E	A question where a little lateral thinking will prove worthwhile – the clue is in the word 'packed'.
Q75	A	A – all statements correct.
Q76	C	Statement 1: True – the description can be verbal as well as in writing, and can include advertisements.

Table 5.4 (*continued*)

Question number	Answer code	Reason
		Statement 2: False – 'trade' includes a retailer, wholesaler and manufacturer; the wider term business is thought to include professions too.
Q77	B	Statement 1: True – for example, it would be a contravention of the Act to claim that a shampoo had not been tested on animals when it had, as this would be deemed to be part of the production process. Statement 2: True – not an explanation but a separate statement.
Q78	C	Statement 1: True. Statement 2: False.
Q79	A	Although it has been reformulated, Nylax is still listed as a laxative particularly liable to abuse in the Medicines, Ethics and Practice guide.
Q80	C	Again, sedating antihistamines are listed as being liable to abuse, but Dramamine is mentioned specifically.
Q81	D	The pharmacist is obviously concerned for the wellbeing and safety of the patient, but as the prescription was not signed by a doctor registered in the UK, it is an illegal supply.
Q82	D	The Medicines Act has been amended to classify paracetamol tablets as POM, except under certain conditions. For non-effervescent tablets for an adult, with a maximum strength of 500 mg, the maximum amount that can be sold is 100. An ethical consideration has no doubt been made, but the sale is illegal.
Q83	C	No contravention of the Medicines Act has taken place, as the pharmacist is selling them himself; he is also well aware of Practice guidance concerning substances of misuse.
Q84	B	It is not legal, as the pharmacy will no longer be under the personal control of the pharmacist, so that even the medicines classified as GSL cannot legally be sold, under the provision of the Medicines Act. The action is not ethical either, as the terminally ill patient will be without their medication.
Q85	E	They are known as Koplik's spots.
Q86	A	Although the two diseases are very different, it is often hard to diagnose German measles, so the appearance of swollen glands at the back of the head is very helpful.
Q87	C	A difficult choice – you might well think the answer would be what his mother thinks, after all he isn't her first baby. The overriding factor is the age of the baby – 8 weeks old, and that he's not feeding – potentially very serious in such a young baby.
Q88	D	For a healthy adult, a few days' illness not really significant; but she is in pain, which is difficult to describe to another – look for clues re pallor, stance etc. She is not in an obvious danger group EXCEPT female, child-bearing age. It could be an ectopic pregnancy, and it certainly doesn't sound like 'flu.
Q89	D	Although all the information is very interesting, it's also relevant. The customer is not really ill – yet. He is a regular traveller to undeveloped countries, and obviously knows the dangers, so that's the overriding factor, but is not listed.

continued overleaf

Table 5.4 (continued)

Question number	Answer code	Reason
Q90	E	There's a bit of psychology here – what's behind the very simple request? Is it that the mother cannot talk to her daughter about what is happening to her? Perhaps an opportunity to open up a dialogue, before she gets to the teenage years.
Q91	A	She appears to have had an infection, and has seen the doctor. She needs to return reasonably soon; you cannot sell her anything effective and the doctor needs to know that the problem has not been resolved.
Q92	B	This could be acute glaucoma, which is a medical emergency and needs treating a.s.a.p.
Q93	C	All the signs of hayfever; there's no reason, e.g. pregnancy, not to sell her an appropriate remedy.
Q94	D	Following the 'RICE' advice for such injuries, suggest an ice pack – he's doing all the rest already.
Q95	D	The only sign that the sting has caused problems is number 1; the others are to be expected as a result of the sting.
Q96	B	As Loperamide is not licensed for sale, the only other answers are 1 and 2.
Q97	B	More complex but the outcome is the same: if she is to have loperamide in addition to the codeine, the doctor will have to prescribe it.
Q98	A	As they are both healthy, and well aware of the possible dangers, there doesn't seem any reason why they shouldn't have loperamide. Might be as well to just check for possible pregnancy though.
Q99	E	For Questions 99–101, check the sources indicated by the answer code.
Q100	C	
Q101	D	
Q102	D	Knowledge; for Questions 102–107, check the BNF.
Q103	C	
Q104	C	
Q105	C	
Q106	E	
Q107	B	
Q108	E	All that is needed is common sense; read all the information carefully. Long-term medication in children should always be sugar-free preparations whenever possible to avoid dental caries.
Q109	C	As she is vomiting, she won't be able to benefit from oral preparations.
Q110	D	A liquid is better if she cannot swallow; there is no need for it to be sugar-free as the course will only be short, and the taste is important to encourage compliance.
Q111	B	For Questions 111–117, knowledge at a fairly basic level.
Q112	D	

Table 5.4 (*continued*)

Question number	Answer code	Reason
Q113	C	
Q114	E	
Q115	D	
Q116	B	
Q117	E	
Q118	D	For Questions 118–120, refer to *Pharmaceutical Practice* Chapter 22.
Q119	E	
Q120	C	

5.5.2 Analysis of skill and level of difficulty of sample questions

See Table 5.5 for analysis of skills and level of difficulty.

Table 5.5 Analysis of skills and level of difficulty
Skills being tested K = knowledge C = comprehension A = application
E = analysis/evaluation
Level of difficulty H = hard A = average E = easy

Question number	Skill being tested	Level of difficulty
Q1	C	E
Q2	C	E
Q3	C	E
Q4	C	E
Q5	E	A
Q6	E	H
Q7	C	E
Q8	C	E
Q9	E	H
Q10	E	H
Q11	A	A
Q12	A	A
Q13	E	H
Q14	E	H

continued overleaf

Table 5.5 (*continued*)
Skills being tested K = knowledge C = comprehension A = application
E = analysis/evaluation
Level of difficulty H = hard A = average E = easy

Question number	Skill being tested	Level of difficulty
Q15	E	H
Q16	E	H
Q17	E	H
Q18	C	A
Q19	E	A
Q20	E	H
Q21	E	H
Q22	E	H
Q23	E	H
Q24	E	H
Q25	E	H
Q26	E	H
Q27	E	H
Q28	E	H
Q29	E	H
Q30	E	H
Q31	A	E
Q32	A	E
Q33	A	H
Q34	A	H
Q35	C	E
Q36	C	A
Q37	C	A
Q38	C	A
Q39	C	A
Q40	E	A
Q41	E	A
Q42	E	A
Q43	E	A
Q44	E	A

Table 5.5 (*continued*)
Skills being tested K = knowledge C = comprehension A = application
E = analysis/evaluation
Level of difficulty H = hard A = average E = easy

Question number	Skill being tested	Level of difficulty
Q45	E	A
Q46	E	A
Q47	E	A
Q48	E	A
Q49	E	A
Q50	E	A
Q51	E	A
Q52	E	A
Q53	E	A
Q54	A	A
Q55	A	A
Q56	A	A
Q57	A	A
Q58	A	A
Q59	A	A
Q60	A	A
Q61	A	A
Q62	A	A
Q63	A	A
Q64	A	A
Q65	A	A
Q66	A	E
Q67	A	E
Q68	A	E
Q69	A	E
Q70	K	E
Q71	K	E
Q72	K	E
Q73	C	A
Q74	C	A

continued overleaf

Table 5.5   (*continued*)
Skills being tested K = knowledge C = comprehension A = application
E = analysis/evaluation
Level of difficulty H = hard A = average E = easy

Question number	Skill being tested	Level of difficulty
Q75	K	H
Q76	K	H
Q77	E	H
Q78	C	H
Q79	K	E
Q80	K	E
Q81	E	H
Q82	E	H
Q83	E	H
Q84	E	H
Q85	K	A
Q86	K	A
Q87	A	H
Q88	A	H
Q89	A	H
Q90	A	H
Q91	A	E
Q92	A	H
Q93	A	H
Q94	A	H
Q95	K	E
Q96	C	E
Q97	A	A
Q98	C	E
Q99	E	A
Q100	E	A
Q101	E	A
Q102	K	A
Q103	K	A
Q104	K	A

Table 5.5   (*continued*)
Skills being tested K = knowledge C = comprehension A = application
E = analysis/evaluation
Level of difficulty H = hard A = average E = easy

Question number	Skill being tested	Level of difficulty
Q105	K	A
Q106	K	A
Q107	K	A
Q108	C	E
Q109	C	A
Q110	C	A
Q111	K	A
Q112	K	A
Q113	K	A
Q114	K	E
Q115	K	E
Q116	K	E
Q117	K	E
Q118	K	E
Q119	K	E
Q120	K	E

6

After the exam

Well, that's it – your fate is sealed. The computer will be reading the mark sheets, the outcomes of which will be sent in due course to the Board of Examiners for consideration. Any mitigating circumstances and borderline candidates will be considered, but on the whole there's very little you can do – except of course worry about the outcome. You could spend some time reflecting on all the achievements of the past year, and the progress that you have made since graduating (except for Bradford and other sandwich students!), but realistically, all anyone can ever think about is their result.

As with every life event for which there is a long build-up and much planning, everything that happens immediately afterwards tends to be an anti-climax. The period after the registration exam is likely to be even worse; you have probably got to go back to work, complete various tasks, prepare to leave, and there is of course the constant worry of what the outcome will be. The natural reaction is to concentrate on all the 'worst-case scenarios' and not to think positively about what you will do after you receive the coveted letter. Apart from the obvious, such as taking any remaining holiday entitlement, there is another activity where your time could be used constructively.

Even if you are able, or sensible enough, to think positively, it's very tempting to think only about the immediate future after qualifying, and not the longer-term plans that, as a professional person, you should be making. Assuming that you agree that *any* activity is infinitely preferable to the miserable preoccupation enforced on you for the next three weeks, there are lots of ideas you might like to consider. What you actually do will, of course, depend very much on your immediate career plans, but it's never too soon to consider the options that will be open to you, once qualified.

There is one thing in particular that all pharmacists need to do as a major professional obligation – namely to keep to their key responsibility of keeping up to date, as encompassed in the *Code of Ethics*.

The intention of this very short final chapter, which will hopefully be read immediately after the exam, is to outline how you, as a newly qualified pharmacist, could start as you mean to go on. The past year has largely been spent consolidating the learning that happens in the workplace; the idea now – and for the rest of your professional life – is to continue with that philosophy, but also to go further and anticipate what you need to do to develop *your* particular practice. No doubt you have heard the term continuing professional development (CPD). After all, an understanding of what it means was on the exam syllabus, and hopefully you have seen how it works in action, as it is already a professional responsibility to undertake 30 hours a year of continuing education (CE). Perhaps this is a good point at which to explain the difference in the two terms, as many pharmacists are still a bit confused. Basically, the analogy is a bit like buses and transport. All buses (CE) are a form of transport, but every form of transport (CPD) is not a bus. The buses are geared to the needs of the majority and follow a strict timetable (allegedly) whereas some forms of transport are very individual, just like a car, and are more flexible to suit the occasion or the individual better. One of the very first activities your preregistration tutor undertakes is to evaluate his/her previous experiences as a developer of others and to perform a self-assessment of the tutor competencies – a vital stage of the CPD Good Practice cycle (see MEP). As a result of that exercise, each tutor will probably identify different developmental needs, which might well include standard continuing education material, but could also encompass mentoring skills and time management, for example.

So, where are you going to start your CPD? There's one thing for sure, you won't be alone. The RPSGB, the NPA, all the major employers and many other organisations and individuals have been working for some time to ensure that when the requirement for health professionals to undertake CPD as a requirement of continued registration becomes mandatory, a framework is in place. Its main function will be to ensure that pharmacists are supported in all the stages outlined in the good practice cycle, and will no doubt encourage the use of the portfolios that are already available in which to record CPD.

Enough of the conjecture and theoretical meaning of what CPD might mean and what is imminent – application to practice is much easier to identify with. Consider the following scenarios that you might encounter as a newly qualified pharmacist; for each one, try to think of an activity that would help you to meet the challenge outlined. You could also identify any resources that you know about that will help, and then try to decide if they are CE or CPD if you are really desperate for a cognitive exercise.

(a)   You are going to work at a pharmacy that provides a service to residential homes and does domiciliary visits; where do you start to identify your development needs?

Suggested answer: Order the appropriate CPPE distance learning packages.

(b)   Your new pharmacy operates a needle-exchange scheme and provides a supervised methadone service for drug misusers. Where do you begin to find out what safety precautions must be in place for the staff?

Suggested answer: You arrange to visit another pharmacist who already provides such a service to find out about safety procedures for your staff.

(c)   Your new boss suggests that you should do a postgraduate diploma. You think it might be a bit early to consider such a commitment, but recognise that every other pharmacist in the department has a formal qualification and you don't want to be left out.

Suggested answer: explain your misgivings, and ask if you could begin to find out about the courses that are available in three months time.

(d) The local Primary Care Trust needs to employ a pharmacist as a pharmaceutical advisor on a sessional basis, and is prepared to consider a newly qualified pharmacist with a special interest in the care of the elderly. How do you prepare for the interview?

Suggested answer: A bit of research is needed here – perhaps a literature search of recent Journal articles might help, and should point you towards recent the NHS documents concerning proposals for medicines management for the older person.

(e) The local practice is setting up a new repeat prescribing service and would like to consider how the prescriptions will be transmitted electronically as soon as possible. Your IT skills are limited, but you realise that this is an opportunity not to be missed.

Suggested answer: Most people readily admit to having limited skills – and only acquiring new ones on a 'need to know' basis – this is probably one of those occasions. Show that you're keen to learn but don't waste time undertaking an inappropriate course. The sort of things you will need to know are probably difficult to define – it's probably a case of sitting down and having a go with the system when you are not under pressure, and asking when you really get stuck.

All of the above examples serve to illustrate one thing: that the letter saying that you are now a registered pharmacist is only the beginning of your professional career! Remember that the exam tests your abilities at the level of a competent newly qualified pharmacist, not as an experienced practitioner. In order to progress from one to the other, you need to develop skills and gain knowledge. That is certainly achieved by working, in whichever sphere of the profession you find yourself, but your progress will tend to be reactive rather than proactive. That means that you will only go and find out about something new when forced to do so, rather than by planning what you might need to know in advance, and organising the appropriate resources. But how do you decide what to do? Who is going to tell you? Sometimes there is an answer – the RPSGB, the Health Authority or your employer will make a particular course a necessity, but more often (and more appropriately) it is up to you. The formal process by which you can arrive at an informed decision is known as a professional audit; identifying what you need to do to progress as a practitioner is Continuing Professional Development, which may well include Continuing Education. The 'Good Practice Cycle' to be found in the Medicines, Ethics and Practice guide describes the process in more detail. Probably your initial needs will be to complete CPPE continuing education packages and attend specific workshops, but later on your development will include membership of specialist groups; an example would be the Academic Pharmacists Group for anyone involved in teaching. Don't forget the list of contact numbers for pharmaceutical organisations in your workbook or manual.

Perhaps the activities described very briefly above are too far away to contemplate – you are still at the stage of 'auditing' your performance as a preregistration trainee. Whatever the immediate concern, may you survive the preregistration year and become an effective, independent registered pharmacist – and continue to develop professionally.

References and other useful publications

Appelbe G E, Wingfield J (2001). *Dale and Appelbe's Pharmacy Law and Ethics*, 7th edn. London: Pharmaceutical Press.

Appelbe G E, Wingfield J, Taylor L M (2002). *Practical Exercises in Pharmacy Law and Ethics*, 2nd edn. London: Pharmaceutical Press.

Blenkinsopp A, Paxton P (1998). *Symptoms in the Pharmacy: A guide to the management of common illness*, 3rd edn. Oxford: Blackwell Scientific Publications.

British National Formulary 43, March 2002. London: British Medical Association and Royal Pharmaceutical Society of Great Britain, 2002. [Published biannually in March and September.]

Drug Tariff. London: The Stationery Office. [Published monthly.]

Edwards C, Stillman P (2000). *Minor Illness or Major Disease? Responding to symptoms in the pharmacy*, 3rd edn. London: Pharmaceutical Press.

Edwards C, Walker R (1999). *Clinical Pharmacy and Therapeutics*, 2nd edn. Edinburgh: Churchill Livingstone.

Greene R J, Harris N D (2000). *Pathology and Therapeutics for Pharmacists*, 2nd edn. London: Pharmaceutical Press.

Mason P (2000). *Nutrition and Dietary Advice in the Pharmacy*, 2nd edn. Oxford: Blackwell Scientific Publications.

Medicines, Ethics and Practice: A guide for pharmacists 25, July 2001. London: Royal Pharmaceutical Society of Great Britain, 2001. [Published biannually in January and July.]

Nathan A (2002). *Non-prescription Medicines*, 2nd edn. London: Pharmaceutical Press.

Sweetman S, ed. (2002). *Martindale: The complete drug reference*, 33rd edn. London: Pharmaceutical Press.

The Pharmaceutical Journal. [Published weekly. The official journal of the Royal Pharmaceutical Society of Great Britain.]

Winfield A J, Richards R M E, eds (1998). *Pharmaceutical Practice*, 2nd edn. Edinburgh: Churchill Livingstone.

Index

Page numbers in *italics* indicate figures, tables and exercises.